Malcolm I.V. Jayson, M.D.
Allan St. J. Dixon, M.D.

Understanding Arthritis and Rheumatism

A Complete Guide to the Problems and Treatment

Preface by Currier McEwen, M.D.

Illustrations by Gary James

G.K.HALL&CO.

Boston, Massachusetts

1976

Library of Congress Cataloging in Publication Data

Jayson, Malcolm.
    Understanding arthritis and rheumatism.

    "Published in large print."
    Includes index.
    1. Arthritis. 2. Rheumatism. 3. Sight-saving
books. I. Dixon, Allan St. John., joint author.
II. Title.
RC933.J34 1976   616.7'2   76-26172
ISBN 0-8161-6424-X

Published in Large Print by arrangement with
Pantheon Books

Set in Photon 18 pt Crown

To Judi and Sheila

Contents

Facts on Arthritis   xi

Arthritis Warning Signs   xiii

Preface, by Currier McEwen, M.D.   xv

Introduction   xxi

1. **Our Shared Inheritance**   1

   The Structure of the Spine   2

   The Causes of Backache   6

   Treatment and Prevention
   of Backache   19

2. **Backache Due to Inflammation, Bone Disease, and Tumors**   41

   Ankylosing Spondylitis   42

   Bacterial Infections of the
   Spine   65

Abnormalities in the
    Development of the Spine   67
Bone Disease   68
Spinal Tumors   74
Referred Pain   76
To Sum Up   77
3. **Neck Pains**   **78**
The Structure of the Neck   78
Cervical Spondylosis   81
Herniated Cervical Disc   85
Cervical Fibrositis   87
Neckache Associated with
    Other Diseases   88
Factors and Conditions
    Relating to Neck Pain   89
The Symptoms of Wear-and-
    Tear Diseases of the Neck   91
Treatment   94
Research into the Neck   101
4. **Rheumatoid Arthritis**   **103**
How Widespread Is It?   104
What Is the Cause?   106
What Happens?   109

Treatment 117

The Outlook for Rheumatoid
Patients 151

5. **Diseases Resembling
Rheumatoid Arthritis** 153

Arthritis and Psoriasis 153

Reiter's Syndrome 158

Ulcerative Colitis and
Regional Enteritis 161

Systemic Lupus Erythematosus
and Other Autoimmune
Diseases 165

Venereal Disease and Arthritis 169

6. **Ageing, Wear and Tear, and
Osteoarthritis** 174

Ageing, or Wear and Tear 175

Osteoarthritis 182

Treatment 188

7. **Gout and Pseudo-Gout** 195

Inflammation Due to Crystals 198

Gout — A Rich Man's Disease? 202

Treatment 212

Pseudo-Gout: Chondrocalcinosis 220

Periarticular Calcification 223

8. **Soft Tissue Rheumatism** 224
Generalized Soft
Tissue Rheumatism 227
Localized Soft Tissue
Rheumatism 233
Treatment 249
Factors Increasing the
Discomfort of
Rheumatism 250

9. **Rheumatism in Children** 256
Aches and Pains 258
Rheumatic Fever 263
Still's Disease (Juvenile
Rheumatoid Arthritis) 271
Rarer Causes of Arthritis
in Children 281
Preventing Arthritis and
Rheumatism in Adult Life 290

10. **Painful Feet** 292
The Anatomy of the Foot 294
Shoes and Foot Deformity 299
Pain in the Foot 308

The Foot in Old Age 315

The Foot in Arthritis 316

The Foot in Diabetes 320

The Foot and Leprosy 322

Treatment 324

11. **Does Arthritis Affect Family Life and Sex Life?** 338

How Rheumatism Affects the Young 339

Planning for and Having a Family 344

Pregnancy and Arthritis 347

Making Love 354

12. **Spas and Spa Therapy** 361

The Development of Spas 361

Spa Treatments 367

The Decline of the Old Spa 372

13. **Acupuncture, Herbalism, and Folk Medicine** 374

The Search for Help 374

Assessing the Value of Drugs 377

Folk Medicine and Herbalism 381

Out-and-Out Quackery 386

Acupuncture 388

In Conclusion 390

Resource Directory:

Where to Find Help 393

Agencies 393

Benefits 396

Clothing 396

Community Guides 397

Diagnosis, Consultation, and
   Treatment 398

Education, Information, and
   Schools 398

Employment 399

Homebound Services 400

Recreation 400

Rehabilitation 401

Research 401

Self-help Devices and
   Equipment 402

About the Authors 437

Facts on Arthritis*

- An estimated 363 million people, or 10 percent of the world's population, have arthritis.
- Over 50 million Americans have some form of arthritis.
- More than 20 million people in the United States suffer from arthritis so seriously that they need medical care.
- Arthritis strikes one out of every ten Americans, and one out of four families.
- Approximately 3,500,000 Americans are disabled by arthritis.
- Arthritis in its nearly 100 different forms claims 600,000 new victims every year in the United States. It strikes women twice as often as men.
- Over 5 million Americans are victims of rheumatoid arthritis (RA), the most dangerous and crippling form of the disease. Most RA victims are stricken during the 20 to 45 "prime of life" years.
- There are at least 250,000 children in the

* As of January 1976

United States who have juvenile rheumatoid arthritis.

- The annual economic impact of arthritis in the United States totals over $9.2 billion — and is rising at a staggering rate of $1 billion dollars a year.
- Arthritis costs Americans $3.512 billion in lost wages annually. An additional $772 million is lost in income taxes to the federal government.
- Medical care costs for arthritis total $2.931 billion a year. It also costs families nearly another one billion dollars a year in lost homemaker services.
- Almost 15 million working days are lost every year due to arthritis.
- More than $408 million is wasted annually on worthless arthritis "cures" and remedies.
- Less than $20 million a year is spent in the United States on arthritis research. This means that for every dollar spent by legitimate organizations, more than $20 is being spent on useless devices and phony products.

Arthritis Warning Signs

See your doctor if you have
- Persistent pain and sitffness upon arising
- Pain or tenderness in one or more joints
- Swelling in one or more joints
- Recurrence of these symptoms, particularly involving more than one joint
- Noticeable pain and stiffness in the lower back, knees, and other joints
- Tingling sensations in the fingertips, hands, and feet

Preface

Imagine the outcry if everyone in the metropolitan areas of New York, Chicago, and Los Angeles were struck by a serious crippling illness. Yet, just such a multitude — the more than 20 million victims of arthritis and rheumatism scattered throughout the United States — were met for years only with apathy, public and medical. These people lose over 14 million work days of useful employment each year, more than is caused by all strikes and work stoppages combined. But the figures, dramatic as they are, can give little impression of the still greater loss the more crippling forms of these illnesses cause in terms of suffering and frustrated hopes. It has been well said that no other group of diseases brings so much suffering to so many for so long.

It is natural that the patient and his family wish to be informed about the nature of these diseases and it is important that they should be. The primary purpose of this book is to provide this information. But let it be emphasized that this is not a "do it yourself" medical book! It is a well-known adage in the medical world that a physician who takes responsibility for his own care has a fool for a doctor. If that is true for a physician, it is easy to appreciate how foolish, and indeed dangerous, it is for the patient to attempt his own care. But it is very helpful for the patient to have an understanding of his illness, its nature, and its course, so that he can cooperate to greatest advantage with his physician and know what questions to ask.

Arthritis is not a single disease but a general name for a large variety of diseases which affect the joints and related structures. The main concern of a patient reading this book will be, of course, with the particular form of arthritis or rheumatism that affects him. In this sense, *Understanding Arthritis and Rheumatism* is a reference book as well as a general treatise. It is also the most comprehensive book on the subject that I have seen for the nonmedical reader. Many advances have been made in understanding arthritis and rheumatism in recent years, and the authors have very successfully incorporated this new body of information. Dr. Jayson and Dr. Dixon are both highly respected authorities in the field of rheumatology. In addition to scientific knowledge and broad clinical understanding, they bring to this book a sensitivity to patients as people coupled with the happy faculty of being able to explain complicated subjects simply and clearly. Their concern for the day-to-day problems of people who have arthritis is particularly well illustrated by their direct and practical discussion of the ways in which these diseases affect family life and by the useful Resource Directory at the end of the book.

For a great many years the victims of

rheumatic diseases were the forgotten men, women, and children of medicine. Fortunately, they no longer have to stand alone. The efforts of governmental departments and private philanthropic agencies such as The Arthritis Foundation and its chapters throughout the United States have led to steadily growing interest, understanding, and knowledge and to programs of basic and applied research. The Arthritis Foundation is linked to the Pan American League against Rheumatism, which in turn is linked to the International League against Rheumatism. These organizations are designed to spread the benefits of new knowledge and new research into arthritis and rheumatism to the victims of these diseases as rapidly as possible, wherever the new knowledge has arisen. Already much has been gained in new understanding of these diseases and how to cope with them, and one may look forward with hope and confidence to still more important advances through the research of today and tomorrow. These present and future advances can help the individual patient, however, only where the necessary facilities and coordinated programs of care are available. Much still remains to be done to bring these facilities and skills to all patients whatever their circumstances and wherever they may live. This requires the active concern of an informed public who will demand what is needed. By helping to increase their ranks, this book will have contributed an important service.

—Currier McEwen, M.D.

South Harpswell, Maine
May, 1974

Introduction

Why write a whole book on arthritis and rheumatism? Who would want to read about it? The answer is simple: we all get arthritis and rheumatism in some form or another during our lives.

This book is written neither for doctors, nor for hypochondriacs to indulge in self-diagnosis. It is intended to fulfill a very real need for information. Rheumatism is one of the many medical problems in which knowledge and understanding on the part of the patient make a lot of difference. Doctors are busy people; their time has to be spent on giving a correct diagnosis and recommending or prescribing the most suitable treatment. They do not always have time to explain what is being done and why. Many of the simple forms of rheumatism, such as sprains, cramp, or a stiff neck, do not even involve a consultation with the doctor. This book describes what is happening or has happened, and its aim is to give a better understanding of why some things help and other things hinder progress.

However, the reasons for writing a book seldom coincide with the reasons for reading it. Why read about arthritis and rheumatism? Because it is so widespread; because it is a fascinating subject; because some forms of arthritis and rheumatism have been the subject of remarkable advances in medical knowledge in the last few decades — and chiefly because the remaining forms of arthritis still present major social problems with significant implications for all of us.

The word "arthritis" literally means inflammation of a joint. However, it is widely used to cover close to one hundred different conditions that cause aching and pain in joints and connective tissues throughout the body, not all of them necessarily involving inflammation.

"Rheumatism" is a vague word used for unexplained aches and pains in joints and muscles, usually in the limbs or in the back. Even specialists in arthritic and rheumatic diseases don't agree on a precise definition. In Great Britain, for example, people use "rheumatism" to include most forms of arthritis. In the United States the term "rheumatic diseases" is used as the all-inclusive expression; "arthritis" tends to be more limited to diseases involving the joints, whereas "rheumatism" refers to involvement of the connective tissues around and away from the joints themselves.

Sooner or later we will all suffer from some form of rheumatism. Certain forms, such as the stiffening of the spine and neck that occurs progressively with age, are so common that they must be considered almost normal. Indeed, we would be quite surprised if an old man of ninety was as supple as a young man of nineteen. Much of this stiffening process is painless, but there are often episodes in the course of a lifetime that are acutely painful. These are the lumbagos and painful stiff necks of adult life.

If rheumatism of this sort is in fact normal — and it is difficult to think otherwise since similar changes occur in animals, and even the enormous dinosaur in the Museum of Natural History in London shows a similar stiffening in its spine — does it have an evolutionary purpose? The answer is probably Yes. Most features of individual animals throughout the animal kingdom are present because at some time they helped to ensure the survival of the individual or the herd, or the procreation of the species. Man has descended from arboreal and nomadic ancestors. It is easy to see that an inability to climb trees or an inability to keep up with a tribe on the move would quickly rule out older members, who otherwise might continue to dominate the tribal family groups beyond the age of their maximum capacity. Now such activities are obsolete, and it is interesting to speculate whether rheumatism in the elderly still has a function. Perhaps a ninety-year-old laborer or managing director could cause a few problems.

Other intriguing thoughts follow. If we accept rheumatism as normal, then research into the causes and prevention of the normal forms of rheumatism is really research into life itself. Perhaps it is a battle that will never ultimately be won, but even so, there are good reasons for not abandoning the fight. After all, a few lucky people have normal or nearly normal joints and spines throughout old age. In others these structures seem to wear out prematurely or very painfully.

What are the differences between these people? Are they chemical — something to do with the actual composition of the bones and joints themselves? Are they differences in the way the body was originally constructed? Are we all basically the same, but do some of us wear out more quickly from hard work, bad posture, or poor nutrition? Even if research cannot hope to provide us with perfect, lasting joints, we can hope that it will explain how we can get better and longer use of the joints that we actually have.

The joints themselves are fascinating objects for research, although it is only relatively recently that medicine has taken a scientific interest in them. Other systems in the body are more dramatic. Stop the heart or lungs and man dies within minutes. Research into heart or lung disease is much more appealing since it offers an obvious way of saving life. Damage the joints and the sufferer is crippled, but he does not die. Research into joint disease has seemed less important in the past. But today we are learning, through research, how to control inflammation in joints and to replace severely damaged joints by spare-part surgery, just as we can replace kidneys and arteries.

Some of these advances have been so successful that certain diseases are no longer even talked about because they have disappeared. Tuberculous arthritis, for example, along with other kinds of tuberculosis, is practically nonexistent in affluent countries. The reason is simple.

We have learned that this disease is spread by infected milk and so it has been possible to eliminate the sources of infection in milk supplies and to test herds of cows for signs of the disease. Sufferers from the disease can now be cured by new antituberculous antibiotics.

The virtual disappearance of rheumatic fever is another victory. Rheumatic heart disease afflicts an estimated 100,000 children and 1,600,000 adults. But mortality in the United States from rheumatic heart disease has declined sharply in the five-to-twenty-four age group — from 1,074 deaths in 1949 to only 297 in 1968, the last year for which figures are available. Now if it occurs it is usually in one of the mild forms that do not cause any lasting damage. Yet the organism that causes rheumatic fever is still with us. Known as hemolytic streptococcus, it still infects children, causing them to have sore throats. Mysteriously, this is no longer followed by rheumatic fever. Some of the credit must go to antibiotics like penicillin, but much must be due to better public health measures. At the moment we don't know which — clean water, clean food, less overcrowding, better diets — any or all of these may be important. The disease in its old and dangerous form is still present in less affluent areas such as South America and India.

Research has led the way to important medical advances for some arthritic conditions, but there are still more victories to win. Of these, the greatest battle is undoubtedly with rheumatoid arthritis. This is, for many, a crippling form of arthritis. It is also one of the commonest well-defined medical problems for which research has yet to provide cause or cure.

Cancer and heart disease are more prevalent, it is true, but neither of these is just one disease. There are some forms of cancer and heart disease that are now curable. During your own lifetime, you, the reader, will have witnessed the triumphs of medical research in many killing or crippling diseases. Diabetes, pernicious anemia, tuberculosis, syphilis, infantile paralysis (poliomyelitis), and a host of other infections have either disappeared or are treatable. By contrast, rheumatoid arthritis stubbornly remains unsolved.

These medical facts of life are at last being recognized on a national and an international level, and consequently the direction of public health resources is beginning to change. Until now, the main effort of the World Health Organization has been directed against the great killing diseases — infections, heart disease, and cancer. But increasingly it is realized that these are of less economic importance than the great crippling diseases such as arthritis and stroke. Although arthritis does not kill, it may prevent people from working and it does cause them to require medical help and economic aid.

In many countries the organization of the services to help those crippled with arthritic and rheumatic diseases is still in its infancy. Some, however, are able to offer more than others in what they can do for sufferers. Disability is, after all, relative. A man in the middle of Africa is severely disabled if he is shortsighted and has lost his glasses. In the middle of New

York there would be no problem — he could go to any optician and get some more. Similarly, people disabled by rheumatism can lead relatively normal lives in countries where the means and aids are there to help them.

Apart from help given to those already affected, an enormous amount of research is being carried out into such problems as rheumatoid arthritis. Rough calculations show that over $400 million is spent each year throughout the world on research that is directly or indirectly related to this problem. It does not seem possible that the disease can resist research for many more years. Then at last we shall see another great victory in the battle against arthritis and rheumatism.

Understanding Arthritis and Rheumatism

1

Our Shared Inheritance

Backache is one of the curses of man, and as with all curses, a legend has emerged in explanation. The legend relates that, when man the hunter first began to attack and kill the animals of the forest, these creatures arranged a meeting to discuss defensive tactics. Each animal decided to curse man with a disease. The pig, who loved eating, gave him indigestion; the sheep declared that he should live without hair; the horse, that he should walk on two legs only; and the antelope, a graceful runner, that man should get rheumatism in his joints.

But legends aside, backache is both a very old problem and a very common one. Examination of skeletons of ancient Egyptian mummies has provided

1

evidence of problems similar to those of today, and the commonness of backache today must surely be self-evident.

Actual figures show that 50 percent of all adults suffer from attacks of back pain. Every year in the United States, of the 14 million working days lost due to arthritis, the commonest single complaint is backache. The days lost to industry due to arthritis and rheumatism are several times the total number of lost days resulting from strikes and industrial disputes. So, strange as it may sound, back troubles play an important part in the national economy.

THE STRUCTURE OF THE SPINE

The fact that so many different problems emerge from the back is not surprising when considered in relation to the structure of the spine. It has to bear the weight of the body and yet be capable of bending and straightening for many years — such a construction would be considered a superb engineering achievement. The upright posture throws

2

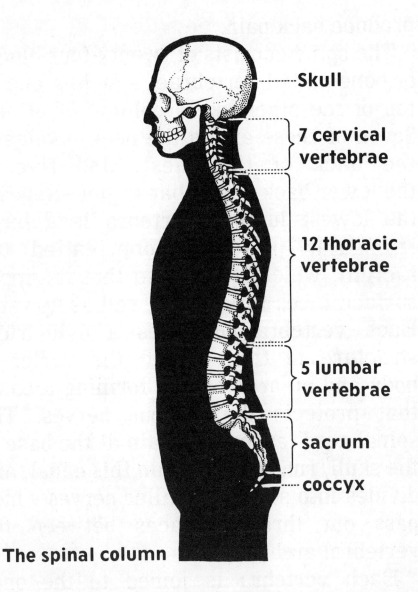

Skull

7 cervical vertebrae

12 thoracic vertebrae

5 lumbar vertebrae

sacrum

coccyx

The spinal column

enormous strains on the spinal column and its associated ligaments and tendons.

The spine is a very complex structure and the principles of its construction must be visualized clearly in order to understand the various problems that

3

produce back pain.

The spine consists of twenty-four blocks of bone called vertebrae, standing one on top of the other like a column of bricks. Seven of these are in the neck, twelve in the back of the chest, and five in the lower back or lumbar region. Beneath the lowest lumbar vertebra is a large triangular plate of bone called the sacrum, which is tilted so that its upper surface faces forward as well as upward. Each vertebra possesses a cylindrical structure in front called the vertebral body and an arch behind forming a canal that protects the various nerves. The spinal cord leaves the brain at the base of the skull, runs down within this canal, and divides into several smaller nerves which pass out through spaces between the vertebral arches.

Each vertebra is joined to the ones above and below by intervertebral discs and by joints. The disc is flat and coin-shaped, acting as a cushion, softening the impact of shocks and jolts through the spinal column. It has a soft, gelatinous center called the nucleus pulposus, and

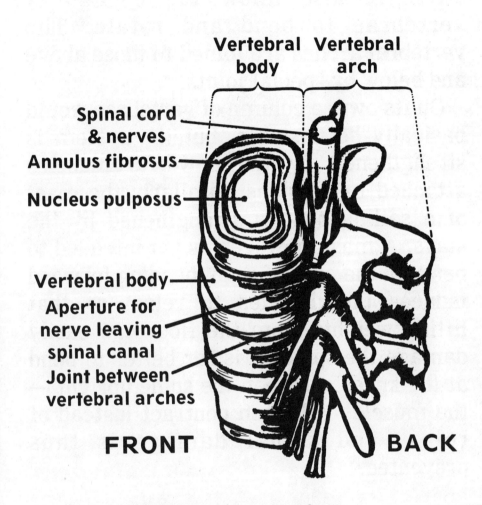

Vertebral body ⎤⎴⎡ **Vertebral arch**

Spinal cord & nerves

Annulus fibrosus

Nucleus pulposus

Vertebral body

Aperture for nerve leaving spinal canal

Joint between vertebral arches

FRONT   **BACK**

Typical lumbar vertebrae

5

around the edge is a layer of thick, tough fibers called the annulus fibrosus. These discs, despite having tremendous strength, also allow the column of vertebrae to bend and rotate. The vertebral arches are joined to those above and below by special joints.

On its own, a column of vertebrae would basically be unstable, but the system is strengthened by the powerful muscles attached to its sides. Similarly the mast of a sailing boat is strengthened by the stays. A mast, however, is not intended to bend. In the case of man, bending forward induces the muscles to relax, so that lifting weights from the floor can easily damage the spine. It is far better to bend at the knees and keep the spine upright — the muscles will then contract instead of relax, and spinal damage is thus prevented.

THE CAUSES OF BACKACHE

Backache is usually caused by problems arising directly within the spine. These are of four main types:

1. Structural change. This can be a sudden mechanical problem, as in a herniated intervertebral disc (commonly known as a slipped disc), or it can result from wear and tear. Also, occasionally, people are born with certain mechanical abnormalities of the spine.

2. Inflammatory disease.* Inflammation can occur in the spine and may affect the joints in a way somewhat analogous to that of rheumatoid arthritis, or it may be the result of an infection and be comparable to an abscess elsewhere.

3. Bone disease.* The structure of the bone may be weakened and give rise to back pain.

4. Tumors.* Growths of various sorts may occasionally occur in the spine and cause spinal damage and pain.

Most backaches, however, are due to mechanical change in the spine (first category), and it is these that will be dealt with in this chapter.

---

* Categories 2, 3, and 4 are all dealt with in the next chapter.

Herniated Intervertebral Disc (Slipped Disc)

As described above, the intervertebral disc was shown to confer tremendous strength on the spinal column. This is true but, under certain circumstances, the central gelatinous nucleus pulposus may burst through the annulus fibrosus. This causes the condition generally known as a slipped disc, but is correctly called a herniated nucleus pulposus or, for short, a herniated disc. The distinction here between terms is significant. A slipped disc, the phrase with which we are so familiar, creates the wrong impression, for it suggests that the whole disc slips and could perhaps slip back again into position. These implications obscure the actual situation — which is that the center of the disc has burst through the outer ring.

Who is affected? Herniation of an intervertebral disc is most common in people between twenty and forty years old. The reason is that at this age the nucleus is most fluid. Later the central nucleus pulposus begins to dry up, becoming tough and fibrous and therefore less likely to extrude.

And yet another inequality reveals itself between the sexes — herniated disc is more common in men than women. This difference, however, is not inherent in the backbones of male and female, but simply reflects the tendency in this society for men to undertake heavier manual work.

What happens? The herniation usually occurs at a weak point in the

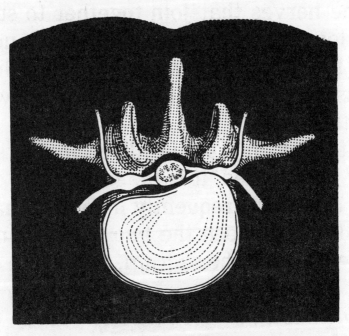

A herniated disc trapping a nerve

annulus fibrosus. This is commonly at the back of the disc toward one side or the other. When it happens, the disc contents are liable to press on one of the nerves that leave the spinal canal. The nerves may merely be irritated or they may suffer more severe damage, but the net result is pain in the area which that nerve supplies. Therefore although the pain originates in the low back or lumbar region — and is felt there first — if one of the nerves to a lower limb is pressed on, then the pain can also spread as far as the foot.

The nerves that join together to supply the lower limbs form the sciatic nerve, and it is for this reason that pain due to pressure on the sciatic nerve is known as sciatica.

Although any of the discs in the spine may be affected, it is the lowest two discs that are most frequently involved, that is, the discs between the two lowest lumbar vertebrae and the sacrum.

And why? Herniation of a disc usually occurs after strenuous exercise.

The typical victim is the office worker who lives a soft life all week, sitting at a desk or in an armchair and traveling by car or train every day. Then the weekend comes and he attacks the garden or the house, and an exhilarating game of tennis or golf is exchanged for previously nonactive pastimes, such as reading the newspaper with his feet up. In other words, it is the unaccustomed exercise that initiates intervertebral disc herniation.

The onset The pain that is felt at the site of the disc protrusion is usually intense and sudden in onset. The sufferer feels as if he had been struck in the back but is unable to straighten up and look around. In Germany such attacks have earned the name *Hexenschuss,* which translated means "witch's blow." The idea is that a witch has just stuck a pin into a wax model of the sufferer, who, by sympathetic magic, feels a sudden pain in the back. Yet when he looks around no one is there. The pain may be so sudden and severe that the sufferer goes pale and may faint.

When one of the nerves is directly compressed, the pain spreads down the legs and sciatica develops — this usually appears within a few hours. The exact site of the pain depends upon which particular nerve is affected. Numbness or tingling may also develop in the area of skin supplied by the nerve while the muscles that the nerves supply may be weakened. Other ligaments in the spine can also be irritated and produce pain. This is felt as a persistent dull ache over the whole of the lower back and also in the legs.

The symptoms Patients with a herniated intervertebral disc not only suffer from great pain but are also unfortunate enough to resemble a rather stiff wooden puppet in their somewhat restricted movements. The difficulty in moving about and in bending the spine is created by the muscles in the back strongly contracting. This is an automatic attempt by the body to reduce the pressure of the herniated disc on the spinal nerves. Raising the leg by bending the hip and keeping the knee straight stretches the spinal nerves and aggravates the pain.

The doctor examines the patient to discover the areas of skin where there is loss of feeling and the muscles that have become too weak to show normal reflexes. All these changes reflect damage to the nerves and their consequent failure to function properly. The information collected will often enable the doctor to locate the exact disc that is at fault.

And the after-effects Ninety percent of all attacks clear up after a few weeks of complete bed rest. The pain and limitation of movement disappear while the damaged nerves gradually recover. However, the intervertebral disc has been permanently damaged and is very liable to protrude again and cause further trouble. For this reason, it is important to be careful not to overstrain the spine again. Heavy lifting should be planned in terms of the best and safest way — above all, weights should NOT be lifted by bending the spine forward.

Frequent relapses of a herniated disc are by no means uncommon. In time these will gradually diminish but, with permanent damage to the disc, the sufferer may be left with persistent backache.

Degenerative Disease of the Spine (Lumbar Spondylosis)

When the young begin to age Any movable joint — human or mechanical — is liable to suffer from wear. Most automobile engines are discarded after only ten years because they are worn out, but a human joint is less simple to replace, and therefore has to last for many years.

Wear and tear of the lower spine is an example of a degenerative disease that occurs in all of us. Its medical name is lumbar spondylosis. Changes can be detected at the early age of twenty-five — and after that our spines can only deteriorate. Contemplation of this fact incites the imagination to visualize a world full of people with crooked spines and half-functioning limbs. It is reassuring to know that fortunately many of these changes do not produce significant problems and if they do, then their effects are usually temporary.

The sufferers Nevertheless some people, particularly those manual laborers whose work involves heavy lifting, can become considerably — or significantly — disabled. For example, coal miners and longshoremen are more liable to develop lumbar spondylosis than office workers because of the strenuous nature of their work. Furthermore, white collar workers can continue their work despite back problems, but the same condition would incapacitate a manual laborer whose performance depends on the physical effort that he can produce.

What is lumbar spondylosis? In this type of degenerative disease, wear and tear can affect both the intervertebral disc and the joints between the vertebral arches. The change is similar in both areas. Degeneration of

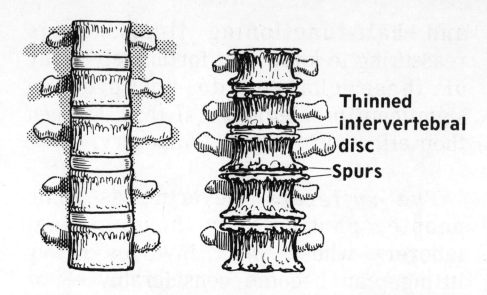

Thinned
intervertebral
disc

Spurs

A normal mobile spine and a stiff spondylitic spine

the intervertebral discs leads to their shrinkage and stiffening. If many discs shrink, the total body height is also reduced, so that old men are often one to two centimeters (approximately two- to four-fifths inches) shorter than they were in youth. Around each degenerated disc, the neighboring bone grows to form outgrowths or "spurs" that may even join up, in extreme cases, to form a rigid bridge between two vertebral bodies. The slippery cartilage that lines the small joints between the vertebral arches becomes damaged also, so that the surfaces of the bone become roughened

16

and similar spurs of bone grow out from the side of the joint. Here again, these spurs develop as a sort of misguided effort by the joint at healing, but prevent the joint from moving through its full range. This helps to minimize the risk of further damage, but of course the loss of the normal range of movement — plus increased friction due to the roughened bone surface — means that the spine becomes relatively stiff.

Low backache Lumbar spondylosis is a frequent cause of recurrent low back pain and backache. A persistent, dull aching pain develops which is usually relieved by rest or by sitting upright with the back supported, and made worse by slouching in a chair or by doing heavy manual work. Occasional severe attacks of pain occur, particularly after sudden exercise. The movements of the spine become stiff and restricted, and unfortunately people with this type of backache often have persistent and recurrent back pain.

Fibrositis or Nonspecific Back Pain

Many people suffering from persistent backache are able to move quite freely, demonstrating a full range of movement of the spine. The pain is often increased by poor posture when standing, or when sitting in a badly designed seat — such as those found in most modern cars. There may be tender nodules in the back, and pressure on these aggravates the pain. X-ray of the spine appears completely, or almost completely, normal.

Doctors use a wide selection of names for this condition, such as fibrositis, postural backache, ligamentous strain, lumbosacral strain, sacroiliac strain, and so on. To be honest, these conditions are not understood at all and these names are largely derived from guesswork. There may perhaps be degenerative changes in the spine that cannot be detected by X-rays or any other investigative method currently available. Meanwhile, until research reveals the mysterious cause — or causes — of these conditions, it would seem preferable to be truthful and call them all nonspecific back pain.

TREATMENT AND PREVENTION OF BACKACHE

There are many important points in the treatment of backache. The procedures used depend mainly on the severity of the pain, the extent of the disability, and the cause of the problem. It is therefore helpful to consider all the aspects of treatment together.

Medicines to Relieve Pain

During the period of severe pain, the doctor will often prescribe strong drugs which may perhaps be given by injection. These are usually effective in relieving the symptoms but may have the additional effect of making the patient sleepy — this is perhaps not such a bad thing if he is confined to bed. However, some of these drugs can be addictive and so should be stopped as soon as possible.

When the pain is less severe, more

commonplace drugs, such as aspirin, indomethacin, phenylbutazone, and others may be used. These medicines will be described in greater detail later, in the chapter on rheumatoid arthritis.

Confinement to Bed

Complete bed rest is essential for sufferers in severe pain from a herniated intervertebral disc. The concept is, of course, totally unappealing, especially for those with active minds and bodies. But boredom is a small price to pay for relief of pain. People often struggle on for weeks or even months with severe backache before eventually accepting this advice. Complete bed rest in this context means lying flat all day, getting up only for meals, washing, and going to the bathroom. Even these concessions are only allowed because they involve less effort than struggling with trays, sponge baths, and bed pans.

Two weeks of rest in bed may be necessary before the symptoms disappear. But with strict adherence to these rules, many acute back problems improve within a few days. The rules can then gradually be relaxed and the patient can slowly return to normal living.

Choosing your bed — and lying on it The type of bed is all-important.

The criterion generally used for choosing a good bed is that it should be as soft as possible. But unfortunately this is misleading — soft beds "give" under the weight of the body and as a result the spine lies in a curved position during the night, aggravating backache. Many people suffer from backache in bed due to this very cause.

A firm orthopedic bed, which has a soft surface and yet provides full support, is the best answer. This is where the quality of a bed is important. A cheap bed has relatively few springs and sags easily, whereas better beds have an increased number of springs which provide firmer support.

But for those of us whose financial situation imposes undesirable restrictions on such activities as buying expensive beds, there is a more economical answer. Placing a board beneath the mattress of the bed is a useful compromise, and despite sounding rather austere, it is in fact quite comfortable. Three-quarter-inch plywood is best as it has no "give" to it and will provide good support. The board should be wide enough to support the full body and, of course, be as long as the sufferer. In double beds a board can be placed under only one half, but as this type of supported bed is not in the least bit uncomfortable, it is perhaps more conjugal for the board to be beneath both partners. Because of the size, two boards — one underneath each half of the mattress — should be used for double beds.

Sleeping as flat as possible with only one pillow will also help. Two or more pillows bend the neck, which in turn distorts the lower spine.

Many people who have been unable to obtain a good night's sleep for years have enjoyed complete relief by using these simple means — and once they have started using beds of this type they use them for life. Even people without backache become aware that they sleep more soundly on a firm bed. An interesting fact to note here is that firm beds are generally used in the United States, but American visitors to Britain often complain of back trouble due to soft beds.

Spinal Supports and Corsets

Some people find it impossible to continue with a prolonged period of bed rest despite severe back pain. For them it is possible to immobilize the spine by use of a plaster-of-Paris jacket. This can only be applied by a skilled doctor or technician. The patient stands upright with the back in a good posture, and the soft plaster is molded around the trunk. The plaster then dries hard and prevents movement of the spine. This is a less satisfactory method of resting the spine than confinement to bed, but nevertheless it is sometimes very useful.

In less serious illness, or if the patient still suffers from persistent mild low backache after the pain has become less severe, a lumbar corset can be of help. For this corset to be of any real value it must be tailored to fit the patient exactly. Those seen advertised in newspapers or magazines are of limited use because they do not provide any rigid support and are not tailored to the individual person. A surgical corset of the required type contains steel strips running up the back. These are formed to the contours of the body and restrict the motion of the lower back to a certain degree.

The attitude that corsets are undignified and clumsy may unfortunately hinder some sufferers from using them, particularly if they have heard that many of these corsets make the patient feel hot, sweaty, and uncomfortable. This is no longer true since canvas corsets with steel stays are used nowadays and are airy and comfortable.

Lumbar corsets should be prescribed by a doctor, the patient measured accurately, and the corset supplied by a proper appliance fitter. Even after this, adjustments to the corsets may still be required to provide a satisfactory and comfortable fit.

The corset should be discarded as soon as possible; otherwise lack of movement may cause the spine to become stiff and the muscles to weaken and waste.

Sitting Still and Suffering

The rigors of an unpleasant sitting position are known to all of us. Many theaters, movie houses, and particularly local auditoriums seem to specialize in agonizingly uncomfortable seats which can convert a few hours of entertainment into an endurance test. This is particularly torturous for the sufferer from back pain.

Certain basic points in the design of the chair must be borne in mind.

The purpose of a chair is of prime consideration. A waiting-room chair in an office does not need to give the same degree of long-term comfort as does the chair of the receptionist. Although even this could be debated when one remembers just how long it is often necessary to wait before being attended to!

In the office The significant point to be made here is that much more attention should be given to the design of office chairs, as office workers spend virtually all of their working lives sitting in them. The height of the chair should allow the knees to be higher than the hips when the feet are flat on the floor. If the chair's height cannot be lowered, a sufficiently thick footrest may be used to bring the knees up. The chair should be designed in relation to the accompanying working surface — it is better to think of the chair and desk as a unit rather than as two separate entities. It is important that the height of the desk be correct. This can be seen when the user rests his elbows on the desk; when his arms are close to his side, his shoulders should not be pushed up nor should he have to learn forward. There should be adequate leg clearance under the desk, and the lighting should be placed in a way that will not force the user to strain forward out of a good sitting position and so nullify the design qualities of the chair.

The comfort of the chair is all important. Comfort, however, is subjectively assessed — the best solution would be individually designed chairs based on personal measurements and seating characteristics. But this is, of course, virtually impossible, and chair manufacturers rely on standard information about the dimensions of the human frame. For office chairs adjustments in height and degree of lumbar support always should be provided.

At home A common misconception surrounding ideas about a good comfortable easy chair at home is that low armchairs with soft cushioning and thick padding are the best, whereas in reality these chairs generate some of the greatest strains on the spine and are the least appropriate for sufferers from back pain. An upright chair with proper support for the low back is in fact very much more comfortable. A small pillow placed behind the low back will often improve the position in an otherwise unsuitable chair. The important thing is to restore the normal hollowing that should be present in the back.

Padding and cushioning of a chair are important in preventing unnecessary pressure on the thighs and buttocks, but too much padding over the front edge can restrict movement and lead to numbness.

And in the car Equal attention must be paid to the design of car seats. These seats, particularly those found in certain small cars, are notorious for initiating problems in the spine. Traveling salesmen are prone to backache because they spend long periods sitting still in a poor position. The ideal car seat should have an appropriate curve to fit the contour of the back and be adjustable so as to provide the most comfortable position.

New developments An interesting point to note is that there are some significant developments in the design of chairs. Every time one sits down on a chair, the spine receives a blow which is softened by thick cushioning. In these new chairs, on the other hand, the padding is considerably thinner but the blow is counteracted by springs in the center column or base of the chair.

The purpose of a chair is to permit one to sit and relax in comfort — and this should be the factor of prime importance when buying chairs. Unfortunately, price, appearance, and durability must also be considered, but they should not be allowed to persuade us to purchase a less comfortable chair.

Drafts and Heat

A need to feel warm has long been associated with old people and rheumatism, and the foundations of this are obvious. Some people are particularly sensitive to the effects of cold, and state that their back troubles are intensified by sitting in a draft. They are unable to sleep at night without a hot water bottle, thick clothes, or an electric heating pad to keep their backs warm. With this particular type of backache a woolen body belt or cummerbund may be beneficial.

Heat is a recognized form of therapy, and warmth to the back is well known for providing a lot of relief. The simplest way of applying heat is by means of a hot water bottle. There is no virtue in this being too hot and certainly no need for it to be so hot as to cause any pain. A comfortable heat is all that is required.

Physical therapists use hydrocollator packs, which are canvas bags filled with silica gel. Silica gel holds the heat for twenty minutes after it is heated in a hot water bath. With proper instruction, the patient can learn to apply such a hot pack himself at home, covering his skin first with thick turkish toweling.

Warmth and heat relieve pain at the time of application, but in general it is unlikely that in the long term they would make any difference to the course of the spinal disease.

Exercises for the Spine

Recurrent attacks of back pain can cause the muscles of the spine to become weakened. Failure of these weak muscles to support the spine properly can in turn lead to the development of further damage. It is therefore important to preserve and restore the strength of these muscles. This is the reason for spinal exercises.

One common feature of all low back exercise programs is that they are aimed at strengthening the abdominal muscles, loosening up tight hip flexors, and increasing the elasticity and strength of the muscles that run up and down the sides of the spinal column. Since exercise programs have to be outlined individually according to the patient's condition, the wisest course is to consult a knowledgeable physician who will have a physical therapist instruct the patient in detail on how to perform the exercises. The physical therapist will gradually increase the complexity of the exercises and the number of times they are repeated, according to the patient's response to them.

It should be stated again (despite the fear of being tedious) that the right and wrong ways to bend must be remembered. When lifting a heavy weight, bend at the knees and keep the spine upright.

Massage and Spinal Traction

Massage is perhaps the most familiar and the most pleasant form of treatment of back pain. Repeated pressures are applied with the side or flat of the hand, softly at first and then with greater force. Massage is applied particularly to muscles in the back that are undergoing painful spasm, and it usually provides temporary relief. Unfortunately, however, the benefit of massage does appear to be only temporary, and when used alone it is of little real value. When massage has been applied to relieve spasm, it should be followed by exercises that produce more permanent benefit.

Spinal traction, on the other hand, does not produce the same pleasant image that massage elicits. Rather, stretching the spine sounds more like the medieval torture rack. Nevertheless, the stretching involved in spinal traction can produce relief.

Originally, this method was applied in order to pull a herniated disc back into its appropriate position. Theoretically this sounds fine, but in practice it has been revealed that it is not possible to pull the disc back in this way. The benefits that the patient obtains from lumbar traction are uncertain except that the patient has to stay in bed — which is likely to be the most beneficial aspect of the treatment.

Spinal traction is applied through a harness with the patient on a frame, but differs from the torture rack in that only small forces are applied, and these are carefully and precisely controlled.

Manipulation

Manipulation of the spine is a very controversial subject. The conditions so far described have all been due to mechanical damage and it would seem that these should be correctible by mechanical means. Undoubtedly some patients improve considerably following manipulation by a skilled operator. However, others are made worse.

The spine is a complex structure containing many delicate structures. Sudden mechanical displacement of two vertebrae can easily damage the internal tissue structures in the spine and may produce permanent and irreversible damage. It is the basic difficulty in distinguishing between patients who will benefit from manipulation and those who might be made worse that is essentially at the center of the whole controversy surrounding this form of treatment.

Manipulation is applied by doctors, physical therapists under medical direction, osteopaths, and chiropractors. All four groups are highly skilled and have the ability to provide relief. However, careful examination of research data has shown that most backaches that are considered suitable for manipulation will get better by themselves within a few weeks. So that, although relief may be obtained sooner with manipulation — perhaps immediately following the treatment — when assessed at the end of two weeks manipulated patients are no better off than those who are not treated by manipulation.

Chiropractors

The training of chiropractors is not along the orthodox lines of conventional medicine. The medical argument is that there is no virtue in being unorthodox — it simply means that many aspects of the subject have not been covered during training. This argument also holds that erroneous ideas about changes in the spine producing back pain can become accepted by the unorthodox without being challenged by critical observers, by dissection at operation, or by postmortem examination.

But to be fair, it should be added that chiropractors have displayed an extreme interest in patients with back pain who have often been neglected by conventional medicine. It is the failure of the medical profession to take a proper interest in this subject that has resulted in people seeking treatment from other sources despite the attendant risks. With the current standards of medical care, manipulation should only be undertaken by a skilled medical practitioner or by a physical therapist under his direction.

Injections

Various forms of injections are sometimes used for the relief of back pain. For example, a direct injection of hydro-cortisone mixed with a local anesthetic can often relieve the tender areas in the back.

Surgery for Herniated Intervertebral Disc

In severe cases of disc herniation, after there has been a failure to respond to the type of treatment previously described, surgery may be necessary. But this is, in fact, very rare. A thorough investigation is required in order to determine the exact site of damage to the disc. The operation exposes the hernia, which is then removed, together with the remains of the disc between the vertebral bodies, so as to prevent any recurrence.

This type of operation may necessitate several weeks away from work and could prevent a manual laborer from ever returning to heavy physical work.

Diet

Backache is not associated with any particular type of food, herbs, or spice. You can, in fact, eat whatever you like — as long as you are not overweight. The logic of this is quite obvious really — being thirty pounds overweight is the equivalent of permanently carrying a suitcase weighing thirty pounds. The excess weight places extra strains on the spine.

But, as most of us know from experience, dieting is easier said than done. Innumerable special diets, from raw eggs to near-starvation, are attempted for a few weeks and then abandoned in favor of less spartan living. It is more sensible and practical to make dieting into part of a way of life. Once one accepts that certain foods are fattening and should always be avoided, then losing weight will be easier and more permanent. Bread, cakes, crackers, sugar, sweets, chocolate, potatoes, and all other carbohydrates should be eaten in restricted quantities. One of the authors has lost twenty pounds in a few months on this sort of dietary regime.

Future Research into Back Pain

Medical knowledge of back troubles is still incomplete. In many cases the exact cause of back pain is not fully understood, and therefore research using many different techniques is needed to reveal the exact abnormality.

It is necessary to evaluate the type and amount of strain associated with normal muscle movements. Mechanical calculations are being made to determine the size and scale of the forces to which the lumbar spine is subject during use; studies are being conducted to discover the mechanical strength of the body tissues. Also, we have yet to find out whether there is any predisposing weakness in some of those people who suffer from spinal disease. The strength of the back depends upon its chemical structure and this in turn must be studied in relation to practical problems.

Of all the rheumatic conditions, back pain is the one for which it is most difficult to test the value of treatments, especially new treatment. The symptoms of back pain come and go, so that any new treatment the sufferer happens to be taking at the time gets the credit (or blame). Doctors concerned with the scientific evaluation of new treatments have worked out methods for getting at the truth despite this natural variability, but these methods are cumbersome, require the cooperation of many sufferers, and are therefore tedious and difficult to put into practice. This is why it is so much easier to make extravagant claims for a new cure which apparently worked in a few sufferers than painstakingly to prove that it will do anything for all the others or even for the same sufferers the next time they get an attack. Yet these careful, painstaking clinical trials are, in the long run, the only way that knowledge of treatment will advance.

2

Backache Due to Inflammation, Bone Disease, and Tumors

Most backaches occur as a result of the sort of problems dealt with in the previous chapter. However, structural changes (such as herniated intervertebral disc, wear-and-tear disease of the spine, or strain of the various ligaments in the back) do not account for all back pains. In this chapter other causes of backache will be discussed. These are:

1. Inflammatory disease such as ankylosing spondylitis
2. Bone disease, infection, and inborn abnormality
3. Tumors

But even this list does not include all the possible causes of backache. In fact, not all back pain is due to problems arising within the spine; sometimes it is a result of disorders elsewhere, even though it is actually felt in the back. This is often termed "referred pain" and is described later in the chapter.

Because backache can be attributed to such a variety of causes, it is important to be examined medically at the onset of any back trouble. The character of the symptoms, the findings of the medical examination, and the study of X-rays and blood tests enable the doctor to distinguish between these different conditions.

ANKYLOSING SPONDYLITIS

Ankylosing spondylitis is a very curious condition. The spine is first affected by backache which leads eventually to stiffening and an inability to bend. Even when the condition is painless — as it often is — it can be exasperating for those afflicted by it, for the spine can become entirely rigid.

Ankylosing spondylitis has a very ancient and royal history. Sir Grafton Elliot Smith in his excavations of the

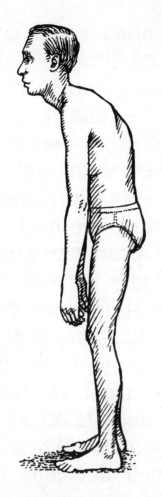

The posture in advanced ankylosing spondylitis

Egyptian mummies in the Valley of the Kings found several skeletons with spines typical of ankylosing spondylitis. In 1741 the Bishop of Cork described a man who was rigid from his head to his ankles. The only job he could do was to be a watchman in a sentry box, because he could only look in one direction and was unable to desert.

Such a description could only relate to ankylosing spondylitis.

Victims of this disease may develop a characteristic — though unfortunate — posture; they may become intensely round-shouldered with such a bent back that looking straight ahead puts a constant strain on the neck. This is rare these days with proper treatment.

If the spine does become rigid but in a good upright posture, then the sufferer is not so badly handicapped; even then, however, he may have difficulty in looking to the right or left. This will interfere with such tasks as crossing the road or driving a car. Worse, however, is when the slouch develops to the stage where, when he is standing, the patient's head is pointing downward to the ground.

From these descriptions it is easy to see how this disease has acquired the alternative name of poker-back. Modern treatment is aimed partly at keeping the spine as mobile as possible but also at preventing a bad posture so that little or no disability will occur.

Who Is Affected?

Ankylosing spondylitis is not an infrequent condition. Statistics reveal that one out of every 330 adult men suffers from it, but (here is yet another advantage for the female sex) in women it occurs only about one-tenth as frequently.

It is unusual in that, unlike most other causes of backache, ankylosing spondylitis affects a young age group. Because the first symptoms normally arise between the ages of fifteen and twenty-five, persistent back troubles that develop at this early age are quite commonly due to ankylosing spondylitis. This is corroborated by army doctors, who find that ankylosing spondylitis is a frequent cause of backache in soldiers.

Recent research indicates a 90 percent or more relationship of ankylosing spondylitis with a certain blood group. In this case, it is not one of the familiar A, B, or O groups associated with the red blood cells (which are important when considering blood transfusions), but one of the less well-known groups associated with the white blood cells. Knowledge of these particular white blood cell groups arose from their importance in correct matching in transplanting organs such as kidneys. The white blood cell group involved in ankylosing spondylitis — HL-A27 — is inherited, so people born with this group, although they do not all get ankylosing spondylitis, have a much greater chance of doing so, 600 times greater in fact. Some physicians believe that an infection in the pelvis is the final trigger in a person who has inherited this susceptibility. There is today a great deal of evidence that this view is correct, since inflammation of the joints of the kind known as Reiter's syndrome, as well as of the spine, as in ankylosing spondylitis, is far more common in people who have this blood group. And it is known that some forms of Reiter's syndrome follow dysentery (inflammation of the large bowel caused by micro-organisms) and others follow venereal disease. The inheritance of the white blood cell groups is closely related to inheritance of the ability to develop certain kinds of immunity both to invading micro-organisms and to one's own tissues. Many people think that inflammatory rheumatic disorders are really disorders of immunity. So research workers have been extremely active in recent years exploring the significance of this observation, which may well prove to be one of the most important discoveries of the decade.

What Happens?

Inflammation The basic change occurring in this disease is inflammation at the site where the ligaments or tendons are joined to the bone. This inflammation then spreads to the joints, and particularly to those in the spine.

The sacrum or tail bone is situated at the base of the spine and is joined to the pelvic girdle by the sacroiliac joints. In ankylosing spondylitis inflammation starts in these joints and gradually spreads up the spine toward the neck. Sometimes other joints, particularly the shoulders, hips, and knees, are affected.

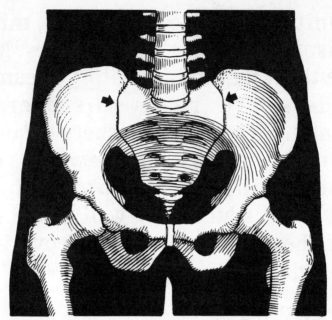

The sacroiliac joints where ankylosing spondylitis begins

A fundamental difference between ankylosing spondylitis and rheumatoid arthritis is in the particular joints involved. In rheumatoid arthritis, inflammation is concentrated in joints in the limbs and rarely affects the lower spine. In ankylosing spondylitis, inflammation is in the spine and does not very often affect the joints in the limbs.

Joint stiffness You might think that inflammation of the spine is an unpleasant enough affliction. However, the real

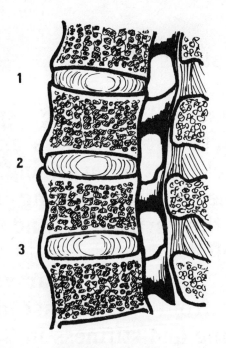

The sequence by which vertebrae become fused

problem is the stiffness that develops as a result.

The site affected is where the fibers surrounding a disc or joint are attached to the bone. Bony outgrowths spread from the edges of the joint into these fibers. They eventually meet and so connect one vertebral body or joint to the next. The result finally is that the joint is no longer able to move. This is what actually happens in many of the spinal joints, and leads to the stiff poker-back characteristic of ankylosing spondylitis.

49

The Symptoms

The onset Ankylosing spondylitis usually starts with stiffness and pain in the low back. But a surprising aspect of this disease is that resting seems to intensify the stiffness and exercise provides relief.

It is very common to hear young men who suffer from this disease describing severe aching and stiffness in their backs during the early hours of the morning. They will often wake at 5:00 or 6:00 A.M. and, as the disease progresses, sometimes even earlier. Their tossing and turning in bed must be disturbing for any unfortunate wives, but it is even worse for the sufferers who are eventually forced to get out of bed in order to perform a few exercises. However, the almost immediate relief gained by getting out of bed and walking about makes such an untimely activity worthwhile.

At this early stage, the spine feels completely normal during the day, and a doctor's examination may reveal nothing unusual. Even an X-ray may not show any changes that could prove which disease the sufferer has.

In a large number of people, the disease comes to a standstill within five years or so, leaving them fit except perhaps for some restriction of back movements. For others, however, the disease progresses.

In more advanced stages of the disease, pain and stiffness persist into the day. Bending the spine is at all times both painful and limited — but this progression is not inevitable for all sufferers.

Sometimes other joints become involved. Inflammation of the hip or knee will lead to pain and swelling and may hinder normal movement.

Severe ankylosing spondylitis Inflammation gradually spreads up the spine and is reflected in the patient's inability to move easily. His movements become so restricted that he finds it difficult as well as painful to bend either forward or sideways, or to twist around. The difficulty — to use a cliché — becomes painfully obvious. Instead of turning his head to look behind, the patient turns his whole body around, and if he needs to pick up an object from the floor, then he is careful to lower himself by bending his knees rather than his spine.

Involvement of other joints has been mentioned repeatedly. When the hips are affected, and if the spine is already stiff, this is a particularly serious complication. It is possible to move around with a stiff spine by using one's hips and knees, and alternatively, with stiff hips one is still capable of many activities using the movement of the spine and knees. But when both hips and spine are affected simultaneously, then the patient becomes severely disabled. Necessary activities, such as sitting in a chair or getting out of bed, can, depending on the exact site of the stiffening, cause immense difficulties.

The joints that connect the ribs to the spine may also be affected. The same restriction of movement in the ribs means that the patient may have difficulty in taking a deep breath. The chest expansion on deep breathing is determined with a tape measure and tells how well the ribs move. In this disease the chest expansion may fall from the normal three inches to one inch or less. Fortunately, we breathe not only with our ribs but also with our diaphragms. In general, the diaphragm can compensate for the poor chest expansion.

Conditions Associated with Ankylosing Spondylitis

Another peculiarity of ankylosing spondylitis is that it is sometimes accompanied by inflammation of other unassociated organs in the body. Nobody knows why this should be — it is just a fact.

The eye In the front of the eye, the iris which surrounds the pupil may become acutely inflamed. The eye feels painful and vision becomes blurred. Iritis, as it is called, occurs in about one-third of ankylosing spondylitic patients; sometimes mild, and at other times severe, it always has a tendency to recur.

Proper treatment is essential in order to prevent damage to the eye.

The heart Occasionally, inflammation may also affect the heart. This is focused around the aortic valve, but fortunately it is quite a rare complication of ankylosing spondylitis.

The function of the aortic valve is to ensure that blood leaving the heart is pumped in the correct direction for distribution around the body. Inflammation in this area may cause the valve to develop a leak and fail to work at full efficiency, so that the functioning of the heart is impaired. In a few rare instances, it may be necessary for a heart surgeon to replace the aortic valve.

The bowels or intestines Finally, revealing even more diversity in the associated effects, certain diseases of the bowels or intestines may also occasionally occur with ankylosing spondylitis. Ulcerative colitis and regional enteritis are two different forms of bowel inflammation producing diarrhea and pain in the abdomen. Both these diseases are causes of inflammation in the pelvis, which in certain susceptible individuals (those who have HL-A27 white blood cell group) may lead to ankylosing spondylitis.

Diagnosis: The Importance of X-Rays

The earliest changes are found in the sacroiliac joints where there are signs of damage, followed by bone spreading across the joint surfaces. Later these bony changes can be seen spreading up the various joints of the spine. Examination of X-rays of the spine is therefore essential for diagnosing early ankylosing spondylitis and revealing how far it has progressed in later disease.

Treatment

Keeping active Physical therapy, spinal exercises, posture: these must be emphasized again and again as being, without doubt, the most important form of treatment for ankylosing spondylitis. Treatment does not just come out of a bottle of tablets or from the tip of a surgeon's knife.

It is only by performing exercises regularly and taking continual care with posture that the mobility of the spine can be maintained and deformity prevented. Infrequently performed physical therapy exercises are not effective — they must be done at least every day for at least a quarter of an hour at a time. Twice a day is better.

The wisdom of this advice, however, does not always generate inspiration in the unenthusiastic. Boredom, lack of time, forgetfulness, and laziness are all used as excuses to justify a lack of commitment, which sadly can lead to restricted spinal movement. Treatment of ankylosing spondylitis is, fundamentally, a constant fight to prevent the stiffening of the spine that characterizes the disease; frequent and regular exercise is the best way in which to fight this condition.

1. The first group of exercises is

designed to maintain the freedom in the lumbar spine:

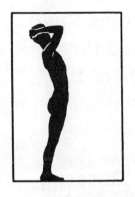

The patient stands with his feet apart, his spine arched backward, with hands above his head.

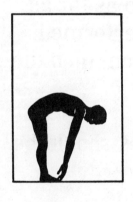

He then bends forward and drops his head downward.

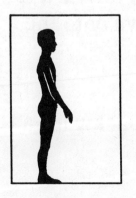

He straightens up, arches backward, and lifts his arms over his head to repeat the sequence.

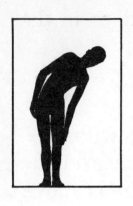

Standing with his feet together, he bends his body to one side, sliding one arm down the outside of his thigh toward the knee, and then bends the other side of the body in the same way.

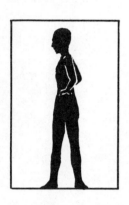

The final exercise for the lumbar spine is to twist the body around so as to point one shoulder backward as far as possible. This is performed first in one direction, then the other.

2. A similar series of exercises should be done for the neck:

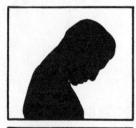

The neck is flexed forward to bring the chin down onto the chest.

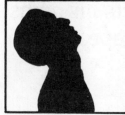

It is then arched backward as far as possible.

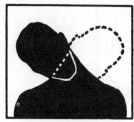 The neck is flexed from side to side, bringing the ear down onto first one shoulder and then the other.

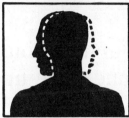 It is then twisted in one direction and then the other, bringing the chin to each shoulder in turn.

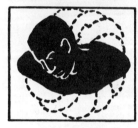 Finally, the head is moved in a circular movement involving all the joints in the neck.

3. Further exercises are designed to maintain the movement of the ribs. These are quite simple. The patient takes a deep breath (using both his diaphragm and his ribs), holds it for a few seconds, and then breathes out again.

4. Exercises for all the other joints of the body have been designed, making use of the full range of movement in each joint.

In particular, exercises for the hips are stressed:

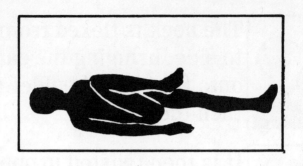

The patient lies flat on a bed and, taking each hip in turn, first bends one knee up onto the chest and then straightens it.

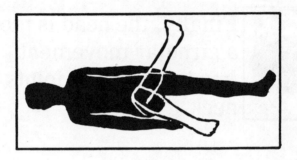

He bends the hip to a right angle and twists the leg outward as far as possible, and then inward.

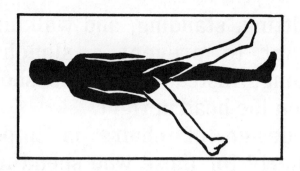

The leg is then placed straight out and the whole lower limb is moved horizontally outward away from the other, and then inward crossing it.

The number of times a patient repeats these exercises should be determined by his physician or physical therapist.

It is important to reiterate that the total period needed to perform all of these exercises is only about fifteen minutes, and, if conscientiously repeated every day, they will prevent most of the trouble that arises in many cases of ankylosing spondylitis. An energetic fifteen minutes each day is indeed a small price to pay for retaining movement in the spine.

Posture The spondylitic patient should always be conscious of his posture when sitting, standing, and walking. It is important to prevent a slouch from developing. Instead the spine should be erect and the head upright.

The design of chairs is important, particularly for those who spend most of their working hours sitting at a desk. Spartan as it may sound, low armchairs should be avoided. An upright chair with some cushioning to support the lower lumbar spine is better.

Beds A common problem already mentioned is the severe early morning aching and stiffness. A board under the mattress (of the same type as is used for people with herniated intervertebral disc) usually provides relief.

Drugs Drugs are of secondary importance in treating this disease. Their main value relates to the exercises — by providing relief from pain, they make it possible to perform the exercises more thoroughly.

Aspirin, indomethacin, and

phenylbutazone are effective,* particularly for relieving early morning stiffness. A large dose of indomethacin taken at night as a suppository may also help relieve the stiffness normally felt first thing in the morning.

Cortisone and other steroids are rarely used for treating ankylosing spondylitis. Apart from not being very effective, they cause other, unwanted reactions.

Radiotherapy or deep X-ray treatment used to be a popular form of therapy, but it has occasionally led to other complications and so it is rarely used now.

Related Diseases?

Sacroiliitis, or inflammation of the joints between the tail bone and the pelvis, is the characteristic feature of ankylosing spondylitis, yet is also associated with other diseases. The problem thus becomes one of definition.

---

* These are described in greater detail in the chapter on rheumatoid arthritis.

Because the changes in the spine are often identical to those in ankylosing spondylitis, it is sometimes difficult to know whether the patient is suffering from ankylosing spondylitis plus the other disease, or whether they are just variations of a single condition.

Ulcerative colitis and regional enteritis have already been mentioned as complicating ankylosing spondylitis. Similarly, it is well known that sacroiliac inflammation may complicate ulcerative colitis and regional enteritis. Hence, it is the old question, which came first? The difference between the two can be semantic.

Psoriasis is a common skin condition in which patches of thickened, red, scaly skin form, particularly over the elbows and knees. Again, spinal changes similar to ankylosing spondylitis develop.

Reiter's syndrome is another quite common form of inflammatory rheumatism. Similar spinal changes often occur in the development of this disease. Reiter's syndrome is sometimes a type of venereal disease.

Finally, Still's disease (which basically is arthritis in children) is sometimes accompanied by sacroiliac inflammation. If Still's disease persists as the child grows up, the final picture is quite often that of ankylosing spondylitis.

These forms of arthritis are all dealt with in more detail in Chapters 5 and 9 of this book.

BACTERIAL INFECTIONS OF THE SPINE

Bacterial infections do not often get into bones, yet bacterial microorganisms can occasionally invade and infect the spine in the same way as any other tissue in the body. Fortunately, such attacks in the spine are very rare but, when they occur, the spine can be severely damaged.

The infection causes inflammation which, when it affects the bone, is called osteomyelitis. If pus forms around the infected area, a spinal abscess will develop.

Severe pain, illness, a high temperature, and shivering are all manifestations of bacterial infections. Tuberculosis (which, mercifully, has now largely been eradicated) is caused by a special bacterium, the tubercle bacillus, usually affecting the lungs, but sometimes involving the bone, particularly the spine. This latter condition has earned the name of Pott's disease — for no other reason than that Sir Percival Pott (1713 - 88) was the first to describe it.

However, the near elimination of tuberculosis means that Pott's disease is currently almost unknown. Bone tuberculosis used to be spread by milk from infected cows. Testing of dairy cattle and pasteurization of milk have been a victory for the public health service.

Brucellosis, or undulant fever, is also an infection transmitted in milk from cows. There is an extensive campaign at the present time to eradicate brucellosis. Unfortunately, this does not seem quite as straightforward as the elimination of tuberculosis. Unpasteurized milk is likely to contain these bacteria; it seems that country living still has its disadvantages, for the risk of catching this infection there is greater. Brucellosis is also common in veterinary surgeons who have to deal with these animals.

The brucellosis bacterial microorganism can become lodged in the spine or in the sacroiliac joints, producing severe pain and spinal damage.

All these different forms of infection are treated with antibiotics.

ABNORMALITIES IN THE DEVELOPMENT OF THE SPINE

Another cause of back pain is related to the complexity of the spine. We expect errors to occur in the building of a complicated artificial structure, so we should not be surprised that abnormalities can occur in the development of such a complex natural structure as the spine.

The many vertebrae of the spine are joined by complicated joints and linked by a system of discs, ligaments, and tendons; it is possible for part of this structure to develop abnormally. For example, instead of five lumbar vertebrae above the sacrum there may be only four, with the fifth one directly or perhaps only partly joined to the sacrum. Alternatively, there may be six lumbar vertebrae, while the sacrum is correspondingly smaller.

These abnormalities are sometimes found when X-rays of the spine are made on people with backache. However, the discovery of an abnormally developed spine is not at all as drastic as it sounds. In fact, it is usually of little consequence — this type of abnormality is found as frequently in people without back trouble as in people with back pains. On the whole, unless they are very severe, these abnormalities of development can safely be ignored.

BONE DISEASE

Bone Structure

Bone is a complicated material. Basically, it consists of an underlying mesh of tough fibers which are strong but lack any rigidity. The apparent rigidity of bone is derived from calcium in the form of a mineral called hydroxyapatite, crystals of which are packed like tiny bricks in this framework of strong fibers. The calcium is originally supplied in our food and reaches the bone from the blood. In order for the calcium to be properly absorbed into the body and manufactured into bones, there must be a sufficient amount of vitamin D. This is the so-called sunshine vitamin, so named not because of any effect that it has but because it is formed directly in the body by the effects of sunshine. It may also be taken in milk, butter, margarine, eggs, and fish liver oils.

Osteoporosis and Osteomalacia

The description of the structure of the bone correctly suggests that weaknesses of the bone are due to two main causes.
1. The first is that there may be a failure in the formation of the fibers forming the framework of the bone. A lack of fibers means that only a limited amount of calcium can be laid down on what is

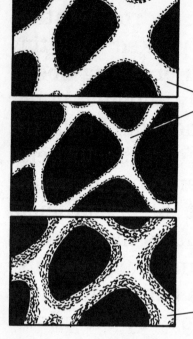

Normal bone framework

Framework
Osteoporosis —
underdeveloped framework

Osteomalacia — normal framework but deficient calcium

Framework normal in bulk but abnormal in calcium

actually there. This condition is known as osteoporosis.

2. On the other hand, there may be a normal amount of underlying framework but an insufficient deposit of calcium. The tissue therefore remains soft and is not converted into proper bone. This condition is called osteomalacia.

Osteoporosis is quite common, especially in elderly people. More frequently seen in women than men, it is the reason for the stoop and loss of height that are characteristic of ageing.

Osteoporosis may also occur as a complication of other diseases and in particular may develop in patients who have been taking cortisone or other steroid drugs.

Osteomalacia tells a rather sadder story. It is due to a deficiency of calcium and vitamin D. In some of our cities the sun is hardly able to penetrate through the smoky atmosphere, so that the body is not able to produce the normal quantity of vitamin D. If this is combined with an inadequate diet, osteomalacia is liable to develop. Again, it is the elderly that frequently suffer. This is because they have a tendency to live on the wrong sort of diet — tea, coffee, bread, and jam — and often do not venture out of doors. At the other end of the scale, young babies in some communities are prone to this condition, although for them the disease involves other special features and is called rickets.

Another reason for calcium deficiency is related to a rather complex chemical in food called phytic acid. This combines with calcium, thus making the calcium unavailable for the bones. Phytic acid is contained in bread, but fortunately is destroyed by yeast during fermentation. However, it persists in the unleavened bread or chapati used in India and in oatmeal porridge (popular in Scotland) and has been responsible for osteomalacia in racial groups accustomed to this sort of diet. A recent experiment in Britain using chapati-free diets for Asian immigrants has led to a noticeable improvement in the amount of calcium available for their bones.

For some people, apparent lack of calcium and vitamin D is caused by a failure to absorb these substances from the bowels. They often appear malnourished, as other nutritious components of the diet are similarly not being absorbed.

If the Bone Is Weak — or the Load Is Heavy

Damage to the spine will occur if the heavy loads it has to support exceed the inherent strength of the bone, particularly if the bone structure is weak. Tiny fractures appear in the substance of the vertebral body, causing sudden back pain. This can be incapacitating and is only relieved after a few weeks when the fracture heals. Recurring fractures of this kind can cause the height of the vertebra to decrease — if this happens to many vertebrae, the sufferer appears to shrink.

Treatment

Only careful examination and blood tests will provide a distinction between osteoporosis and osteomalacia. Any obvious cause is then directly treated. Otherwise calcium and vitamin D are given in carefully measured doses. This therapy is successful in controlling osteomalacia but gives rather unreliable results for osteoporosis.

Acute attacks of pain in these conditions are due to small fractures in the bones. This pain can be relieved by rest. For some it may be sufficient to avoid excessive exertion, although in more severe cases bed rest for a period or a spinal support may be necessary. The difficulty, however, is that rest generates its own problems. Lack of exercise tends to result in the bones becoming even weaker, while using the spine tends to strengthen the bones. It seems to be one of those situations in which you can never really win. A vicious circle can develop: weakness of the bone leads to pain in the spine, which in turn leads to immobilization and further weakening of the bone. Any period of rest for osteoporosis or osteomalacia therefore must be for a strictly limited time. The patient should make every effort to get up on his feet as soon as possible.

SPINAL TUMORS

Spinal tumors are rare, but a brief mention is necessary to complete the picture. They either develop in the spine or spread to the spine from other organs.

The tumors can be of two types. They may be benign, which means that they grow very slowly and can be removed without fear of recurrence. Occasionally they may be malignant. Leukemia and Hodgkin's disease can sometimes affect the spine in this way.

Pain from the tumor is felt in the back and elsewhere, if the pain is "referred." Weakness or loss of sensation may be experienced in the lower part of the body if the spinal cord or nerve roots are damaged. Only careful examination and investigation can determine the existence of a tumor.

Paget's Disease

Sir James Paget (1814 - 99) described a peculiar thickening of the bone which has since been named after him. This, in fact, is not a tumor, but is included here for want of a more pertinent place. The thickened bone has a rich blood supply and can occasionally be extremely painful. New drugs are now being developed that should be of value in controlling this type of pain.

REFERRED PAIN

At the start of this chapter, it was mentioned that not all pains in the back originate from the area in which they are felt. This is due to one of the peculiarities of the anatomy of the nerves in our body. When a particular nerve supplies more than one structure, irritation in one structure may cause pain to be felt in the other. An obvious example is squeezing the "funny bone" of the elbow — this produces pain that spreads into the hand. The explanation for this is simply that the nerve running behind the elbow joint is being squashed.

Similarly, disorders in both the abdomen and the pelvis can produce pain in the back. Such conditions as peptic ulcer, inflammation of the pancreas, and, within the pelvis, various gynecological disorders, may all produce back pain. Normally, however, there are other features or symptoms pointing to the fact that the primary disease does not lie within the spine. For example, with a gynecological disorder the pain is often related to menstrual periods.

TO SUM UP

Most back pains are due to disc disease or wear and tear of the spine. However, there are many other possible causes, most of which have been mentioned in this chapter. Because of these different types of problems, each of which requires a different form of treatment, it is essential to identify the exact cause of the pain.

In conclusion, when backache appears for the first time, medical advice should always be sought.

3

Neck Pains

It is not difficult to surmise how the phrase "pain in the neck" became part of the English language. Both figurative and literal meanings of this phrase describe common intractable problems which frequently occur and which, although not serious, nevertheless produce considerable inconvenience. Neckache is common and troublesome and can affect almost anybody at any age. Although it is usually relatively mild, it can sometimes be both excruciating and disabling.

THE STRUCTURE OF THE NECK

Before describing the different causes and types of neck pain, a brief outline of the structure of the spine in the neck is perhaps necessary to afford a clearer understanding of what can go wrong.

The vertebral column in the neck is similar to the rest of the spine, but differs in that it is designed for greater mobility and flexibility. The neck does not have to support the heavy loads that the lumbar spine must bear.

There are seven cervical (neck) vertebrae; these are all lightly built, and the joints that connect each vertebra to the other allow a relatively wide range of movements. These seven vertebrae stand

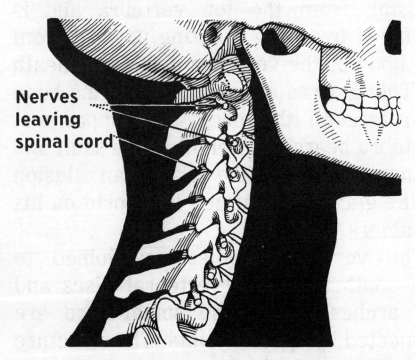

Nerves leaving spinal cord

The bones of the neck

on top of one another forming a column. As with the lumbar vertebrae, each has a large cylindrical area in front called the body of the vertebra and an arch behind that protects the spinal cord. The uppermost cervical vertebra is joined to the base of the skull so that it is in intimate contact with the base of the brain. Between the vertebrae there are small openings through which the nerves pass out from the spinal cord to the limbs.

The two upper cervical vertebrae are more complex. The cylindrical body is missing from the top vertebra and is replaced by a peg pointing upward from the body of the vertebra directly beneath it. This acts as a pivot allowing the head to rotate on the neck. The uppermost vertebra bears the weight of the skull and is therefore called the atlas — an allusion to the giant who carried the world on his shoulders.

The vertebral bodies are joined to one another by intervertebral discs and the arches behind the spinal cord are connected by special joints. The structure of these discs is similar to those in the low back, each consisting of a central gelatinous nucleus pulposus surrounded by a strong tough layer of fibers called the annulus fibrosus. The column of vertebrae is supported by innumerable ligaments and muscles. These impart tremendous strength to the neck while still allowing considerable mobility.

CERVICAL SPONDYLOSIS

Wear and Tear

The most frequent cause of pain and stiffness in the neck is wear and tear of the discs and joints — so-called cervical spondylosis. This is similar to lumbar spondylosis, which was explained in Chapter 1 and is one of the commonest causes of low back pain.

Wear-and-tear changes occur both in the intervertebral disc and in the joints connecting the vertebral arches. The internal structure of the disc becomes deranged and slowly the substance of the disc is lost. The space between the bodies of adjacent vertebrae becomes

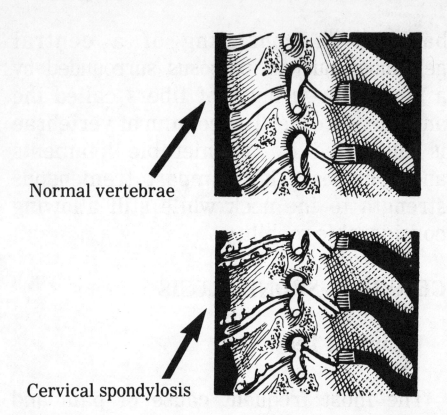

Normal vertebrae

Cervical spondylosis

considerably narrowed and the bone of the vertebra becomes thickened. Bony spurs called osteophytes grow out around the periphery of the vertebral bodies near the intervertebral disc. Similar changes occur in the joints between the vertebral arches.

Stiffness

It is this damage to the joints and the emergence of the bony spurs that restrict the movement of the joints in the neck, with the obvious result that the neck feels stiff.

Pain

Pain may arise in the neck from a variety of causes:

1. Pain may originate directly from the linings of the joints that have been damaged.

2. The various ligaments and tendons may be stretched because of the abnormal stiffness of the spine.

3. The osteophytes that are growing out from the joints may press on some of the nerve roots as they leave the spinal canal. This means that any movement of the neck can easily damage the nerve, producing pain not only in the neck but also in the area that the nerve supplies. As these particular nerves supply the shoulders and arms, it is those parts of the body that are most affected by this type of damage. If the precise site of the pain can be identified, then doctors can usually define which particular nerve root is involved. Nerve damage can produce sensations of numbness and tingling or the muscles can become weakened and lose their reflex responses.

4. In very severe cases of cervical spondylosis the osteophytes project backward behind the intervertebral disc and impinge directly on the spinal cord. This is definitely more than a "pain in the neck," in both meanings of the phrase, for if the spinal cord is damaged there may be weakness and loss of feeling in the whole lower part of the body.

Do We All Suffer?

It is a salutary thought that wear-and-tear changes in the neck begin at about the age of twenty-five and from then on, as with the lumbar spine, the efficiency with which the neck functions gradually decreases. The inevitability of this process suggests that "growing old gracefully" is a wise dictum, as by middle age virtually all spines show some evidence of wearing out.

So cervical spondylosis is very common, affecting almost all adults — it becomes more frequent with the progression of age but usually does not cause severe pain or disability.

HERNIATED CERVICAL DISC

A detailed explanation of a herniated lumbar intervertebral disc — popularly, but misleadingly, known as a slipped disc — was given in Chapter 1. It is also possible, but fortunately rare, for one of the intervertebral discs in the neck to burst or herniate.

Accidents . . .

Accidents — especially car crashes — are the most frequent cause of this type of damage to the discs in the neck. The reason for this is that in most accidents, particularly in head-on collisions, the vehicle is brought to an extremely sudden halt; the driver's (or passenger's) body is held back, perhaps by a seat belt or the steering wheel, but the head is jerked forward by its own momentum. The rapid forward movement is only prevented from continuing by the neck's attachment to the rest of the body, and after a sudden stretching, the head is then rapidly

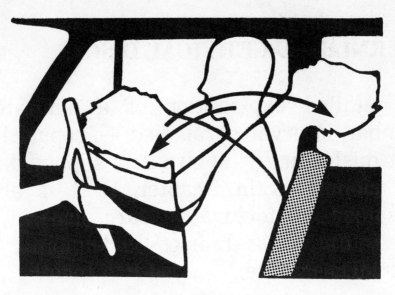

Whiplash neck injury

whipped back, causing the neck to bend backward. The head may oscillate backward and forward in this fashion for two or three times before eventually coming to rest.

Whiplash injuries of this type can produce severe damage in the neck (as well as other parts of the body) and an individual disc may burst in a similar way to that of a herniated lumbar disc. Headrests in cars are a safety measure designed to minimize the risk of this sort of accident.

Herniation of a disc can, however, follow lesser injuries. There may have been some previous abnormality of the disc which, by weakening it, has made it liable to burst.

The burst may occur to one side or the other and directly damage a nerve root; more seriously, the disc may burst directly backward and so damage the spinal cord.

. . . With Unpleasant Consequences

A herniated cervical disc generates severe pain and causes an extremely stiff neck. Sometimes, as a result of this, the neck is tilted to one side.

When the nerve root is damaged, pain, numbness, or tingling may be felt in one of the arms, spreading to the back of the neck and perhaps into the scalp.

CERVICAL FIBROSITIS

Pains in the neck have yet another similarity to pains in the back. This section covers all those instances in which people develop stiff or painful necks that occur for no obvious reason and then disappear after a few days. This condition, termed cervical fibrositis, is entirely analogous to nonspecific back pain* and really just means pain in the neck for which there is no definable cause, nor anything seriously amiss.

In people who appear to be particularly sensitive to the effects of cold and damp, a stiff neck may sometimes develop after sitting in drafts. It is also possible that there has been some strain to the ligaments or the tendons, but neither clinical examinations nor X-rays will reveal any definable damage.

NECKACHE ASSOCIATED WITH OTHER DISEASES

There are several other reasons why pain may develop in the neck, none of which, however, is very common.

Ankylosing spondylitis, for example, can extend all the way up the spine causing pain and stiffness of the neck as

---

* For a description of nonspecific back pain, see Chapter 1.

well as of the back. In some cases, any movement of the neck may eventually be impossible.

Rheumatoid arthritis can also sometimes affect the neck.

Throat infection or inflammation may occasionally spread backward into the neck and produce neck pain.

Tumors of the spine are fortunately rare, but there are various diseases of the nerves that lead to neck pain.

Shingles, or herpes zoster as it is correctly called in medical language, is a painful disease caused by a virus infection that involves the nerves. When the nerves of the neck are affected, it is often difficult to trace the cause of the neck pain until the characteristic rash finally appears.

FACTORS AND CONDITIONS RELATING TO NECK PAIN

The most obvious causes of neck pain are damage within the cervical column, injuries, or any force that evokes a sudden twisting movement of the neck.

Poor posture when standing or too soft a bed for sleeping can also be responsible. Sitting at a desk that is so low or on a chair that is so high that the subject is forced to have his head pointing downward with his neck stretched will, in a few hours, lead to stiffness and aching. Properly designed office furniture should prevent much of this trouble.

Drafts and damp have a peculiar penchant for producing pain and stiffness in the neck. This is a fact that experience will endorse, yet, surprisingly, science cannot explain. A variety of possible causes have been suggested, such as stimulation of various nerves in the neck by the cold or the low barometric pressure, but this seems to be about as far as scientific knowledge has progressed.

THE SYMPTOMS OF WEAR-AND-TEAR DISEASES OF THE NECK

Noisy Joints

A distinctive symptom is a variety of clicking and grating noises that can be heard during movements of the neck. These noises are known medically as crepitus. Despite the rather ominous sounds crepitus itself does not cause pain — although it can be quite unpleasant. It is produced by two roughened surfaces moving against each other.

Chronic Aching

Wear and tear is often accompanied by aching, pain, and stiffness in the neck. The pain is usually of a rather chronic, dull, and persistent nature, although on occasion it may become intensified for brief periods. It often spreads from the neck up into the back of the head or sideways from the neck into the shoulders and down the arm.

Stiffness

The movement of the neck may also be affected. The most marked change is stiffness when bending the neck forward to lower the chin onto the chest. Also stiffness when turning the neck from side to side can be particularly troublesome; this makes such activities as backing a car awkward, for it is difficult to look obliquely backward out of the rear window.

Aching Arms and Shoulders

Earlier in this chapter it was explained that in some people with herniated discs the nerve roots may be affected. This will cause pain to spread from the neck into the shoulder and down the arm. It is a paradox that in some cases there is no neck pain at all; only careful examination by a doctor will reveal the true cause.

Painful Awakenings

Stiff necks are often made worse during the night. Lying a long time in one position (particularly if the neck is bent sharply because of the height of two or three pillows) can be responsible. A soft mattress increases the tendency to awake with a stiff neck because it leads to sagging of the spine under the weight of the body. The sufferer wakes up feeling dreadful and has to wait for some time before the neck gets going again.

Many of these night symptoms can be reduced by sleeping on a firm bed (as was recommended for low back pain) and using only one pillow. There are specially designed pillows with a thin strip down the center so that they are in the form of a butterfly; these allow the neck to lie in line with the rest of the body. You can make one yourself by tying a thin pillow around its middle with a piece of tape; using a baby pillow may be helpful. Or, terrible as it may sound, a bolster or block of wood placed in the nape of the neck may provide the right support.

TREATMENT

Most stiff necks — in fact, as many as 90 percent — will get better without the need of any special medical treatment. All that is necessary is to keep the patient as comfortable as possible.

Heat and Warmth

It was stated earlier that there was no satisfactory scientific explanation for cold and damp having a tendency to increase neck pain. Similarly, it is not understood why warming the neck should provide relief — but it does. Tense, knotted-up muscles seem to relax readily under gentle heat.

Heat can be provided through a variety of methods. Even a simple woolen scarf giving local warmth and heat to the neck will alleviate most stiff necks; a hot water bottle wrapped in a towel and placed at the back of the neck will also help a lot. A silica-gel hot pack that has been inserted in hot water and laid on the neck over thick turkish toweling provides the most effective heat.

Whenever heat is used therapeutically, it should be moist heat, which of course the hot pack provides. The reason for moisture is that it forms an efficient coupling agent to conduct the heat onto the tissues.

Massage

There is no need to explain how soothing and relaxing a gentle massage on the neck and shoulder muscles can be after a tense or busy day at work.

When a patient is in severe pain, the muscles become very tense and rigid, which of course increases his discomfort; skillful massage can relax the muscles and certainly provides considerable relief at the time. But pleasant as this form of treatment might be, in the long run massage does not seem to make much difference to the progress of a painful neck.

Medicine

Because most stiff necks are usually brief and temporary, pain-relieving tablets such as aspirin are used to tide the sufferer over the difficult period. The dosage should not exceed more than two or three tablets taken three or four times a day. If this leads to indigestion or other side effects or if the pain is not adequately controlled, then a doctor must be consulted.

Neck Collars

If the stiffness or pain persists, a tremendous amount of relief can be provided by resting the neck in some sort of special collar. This limits the extent to which the neck can bend or turn and so permits the damaged joints to rest. Usually the symptoms begin to fade after only a few days of wearing the collar, and the problem becomes less severe.

The simplest form of collar can be made by anybody. It is a newspaper folded over, so as to make a strip about three inches wide and eighteen inches long, and wrapped in a scarf. This should be tied around the neck tight enough to limit movement — but not so tight that it strangles the already stricken subject. The result is quite adequate for its purpose.

However, if that sounds too much like the Girl Scout's first aid methods, more sophisticated collars are available from surgical supply houses or can be made for the patient by a physical therapist.

Types of collars
1. The softest collar consists of a thick layer of felt (or a similar type of material) enclosed within a special stocking. This hugs the neck closely and has the extra therapeutic value of providing local warmth to the neck as well as restricting movements.
2. More rigid collars are made of various plastic materials; recently synthetic materials such as fiber glass or plastic have been used, offering more practical advantages than the traditional materials.
3. When it is necessary to wear a collar

for a long period, special types are constructed with padding to prevent the collar from rubbing against the skin, and with perforations to allow the air to circulate so that they do not become too hot and sweaty.

4. All these collars, although differing in their construction, share the same function — limiting the movement of the neck.

Manipulation

Stretching of the neck is sometimes used as a form of treatment. The aim of stretching or traction is to relieve the pressure on the various internal structures of the neck that have been irritated. This is a delicate maneuver which requires a skilled technique and should only be administered by a qualified physician or physical therapist.

Traction can be applied manually by grasping the head and pulling it very carefully in the required direction. Or it can be applied by means of a harness on the head and trunk. It is obvious that extreme care is necessary in order to avoid damaging the internal structures of the neck.

The problems of neck manipulation are exactly the same as with disorders of the low back. Manipulation is applied by doctors, physical therapists, osteopaths, and chiropractors. There is little doubt that skilled manipulation will often rapidly relieve the acutely painful and stiff neck. However, it does not always do so, and sometimes it makes the condition worse. Forceful and sudden movements of the neck can damage the spinal cord or nerve roots with the risk of producing pain, loss of feeling, or muscular weakness in either the arms or the lower part of the body. For this reason some doctors have become rather wary and doubtful as to the true value of this technique. It is impossible to be dogmatic about who is liable to benefit and who to suffer from manipulation, and so it is essential that the patient know that there is a certain risk involved, however small.

Chiropractors have developed special skills for manipulation of the neck. Their fervent belief in the value of manipulation has led them in the past to claim that they could cure not only local problems in the spine but also other diseases such as high blood pressure or asthma. It is the extravagance of these claims that has caused these practitioners to fall into disrepute. It is only at the present time that research is being undertaken aimed at evaluating the techniques of manipulation.

Exercises

After the pain has subsided, the patient may be left with a stiff neck. The answer to this? Exercises. These will help restore the full range of movement, promote the strength of the muscles, break down localized areas of stiffness, and help the neck as a whole to regain its normal function.

A proper exercise program is one that is individually prescribed by the doctor and taught by the physical therapist. As with all exercise programs, the number of times the patient repeats each exercise is gradually increased.

Surgery

The need for surgery for these problems in the neck is extremely rare. A burst disc or an osteophyte in cervical spondylosis may impinge on the spinal cord or on a nerve. An operation may then be needed to relieve the pressure and to prevent permanent damage from developing.

RESEARCH INTO THE NECK

Knowledge of the malfunctioning — and the functioning — of the neck is an area in which the frontiers of science still need to be pushed back. Or to state the problem in a less dramatic way, our understanding of the degenerative diseases of the neck is still relatively poor.

We need to know what initiates wear-and-tear damage in some necks but not in others, and the precise mechanisms by which this damage progresses and gives rise to the common symptoms.

There is a need for more detailed

knowledge of the mechanical changes occurring in the spine during all movements. And, too, the stresses in the different parts of the neck generated during movement have yet to be analyzed.

Treatment of pain in the neck is not based on scientific knowledge, but on methods that practical experience has suggested might be successful. There is a need to understand precisely what it is that provides relief when the neck is manipulated or exercised. And we need to know exactly why local heat will relieve pain, aching, and stiffness. Comparative experiments with different forms of treatment must be applied in order to evaluate which type of treatment is the most beneficial.

4

Rheumatoid Arthritis

The word "arthritis" simply means inflammation of the joints. Rheumatoid arthritis is only one of numerous different kinds of arthritis, and when severe it affects not only the joints but also many others parts of the body.

We are all familiar with inflammation when it attacks the skin and causes such painful conditions as boils — the affected parts become swollen, hot, and painful. When the inflammation clears up, it may leave a scar. Similarly, inflammation can affect the lining of the joints so that they too become hot, swollen, and painful. The joint then becomes difficult to move and does not bend as far as it should. Eventually the joint may be considerably damaged, and internal scarring may stop it from moving freely. Rheumatoid arthritis is the most common cause of inflammation of this type occurring in several joints.

Before describing the symptoms of rheumatoid arthritis, there are four relevant questions to be dealt with:

1. How widespread is it?
2. Whom does it most commonly affect?
3. At what age does it begin?
4. What is the cause of rheumatoid arthritis?

HOW WIDESPREAD IS IT?

Rheumatoid arthritis is a common condition. It affects something like one in every fifty of the adult population. This means that there are over 5 million Americans with the disease, but fortunately most of these people are only mildly affected. Indeed, some have such mild attacks that they do not feel ill enough to see their doctors. They notice temporary pain and swelling in their joints, perhaps in their fingers, but after a few weeks or months the symptoms disappear and there is no further trouble. For others, however, the condition does not settle down, and it is they who seek medical help from their doctor. Of this group, a minority who are more seriously affected develop severe deformities and become crippled. These are the sufferers who are usually referred to a specialist department of a hospital by their doctor.

Who Gets It?

Unlike the conditions dealt with so far in this book, rheumatoid arthritis is much more common in women than in men. For every man affected there are two or three women with the disease. The reason for this difference is not at all clear, but it may have something to do with the female sex chromosomes.

At What Age?

Rheumatoid arthritis usually begins between the ages of twenty and forty-five, but it can start at any age. The disease has been recorded in an infant of only nine months, and at the other extreme of life's span, the condition can develop for the first time in elderly people, even in those over the age of ninety.

WHAT IS THE CAUSE?

The cause of rheumatoid arthritis is still unknown. Scientists have developed a number of theories, and of these there are three that are most generally accepted:

1. The first theory suggests that the body inadvertently alters its defense mechanisms so as to attack its own joint linings — the synovial membranes. This explanation comes from the observation that the joint linings show changes that are similar to those seen in any part of the body in which an antibody reaction is involved in resisting a virus.

To enlarge on this latter point: we are already familiar with the term "immunity." A person is unlikely to suffer more than one attack of measles — because after the first attack the body has developed resistance against the measles virus. This resistance is due to the development of antibodies against the particular infection and to the appearance in the blood of cells that have learned how to attack the invader. Once these changes are present, fresh measle viruses entering the body are immediately killed. The body has developed immunity to measles.

Immunity, therefore, has a very important task in the body. But it can be harmful, or even destructive, in other circumstances. A person suffering from a severe kidney disease may develop similar antibodies against a transplanted kidney and, ironically, his immunity will kill the new kidney in exactly the same way that it kills infecting organisms. This happens even though the kidney is essential for the person's survival.

In rheumatoid arthritis, for some unaccountable reason, the body's defense mechanisms may react against the joint lining in a similar way. The joint lining becomes inflamed and damages the joint.

Although plausible, this theory does not fit all the facts. Immune reactions certainly occur in people with rheumatoid arthritis, but it now appears that they are not the basic cause of the disease. On the other hand, immune reactions assume a greater importance in a rare but related condition called systemic lupus erythematosus, which is dealt with in more detail in the next chapter.

2. A second theory is that rheumatoid arthritis is directly caused by some type of persistent infection. There are a number of known infections in animals in which the invading organisms enter joints to produce inflammation that is similar in some respects to rheumatoid arthritis. Intensive studies are currently being made to determine whether rheumatoid arthritis in man could be due to a persistent infection of this type.

3. The third theory combines the other two. An infection damages the joint so much that the body no longer recognizes it as its own tissues. So it develops antibodies against the damaged joint.

WHAT HAPPENS?

The first noticeable changes — as the previous discussion of its possible causes implies — are swelling and inflammation of the lining of the joint — the synovium or synovial membrane. This becomes abnormally thick and swollen due to persistent inflammation, and eventually it grows and spreads over the surfaces of the joint. If the disease is severe, it can damage the underlying cartilage — which is the natural load-bearing surface of the joint. Eventually it eats its way through, causing irreversible damage to the normal, smooth, slippery joint surface. The ligaments that provide stability to the joint are also weakened, so that not only

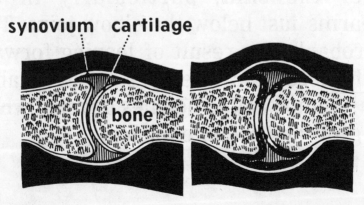

The synovium in normal and rheumatoid joints

is the efficiency of the joint greatly diminished but it also becomes unstable. Damage and pain can ensue because the joint is moved in directions or degrees for which it was not originally designed.

Movements can become so restricted due to the inflammation that the joint will only move through a part of its normal range; this is called a contracture. Or the alignment of the joint can be so disturbed that there is a partial or a full dislocation. In the case of the knees it may happen that the joint bends sideways to produce a knock-knee deformity.

Skin Nodules

Inflammation can also occur in tissues under the skin, particularly in the forearms just below the elbow joint. This is probably the result of leaning forward on the forearms when resting at a table. Small lumps called nodules develop which can grow and become tender.

Not Feeling Well

Although rheumatoid arthritis principally affects the joints, it is important to remember that it is also a generalized disease affecting the total health of the person. This means that there may be changes elsewhere. The subject often feels unwell, tires easily, and is very irritable. He or she is likely to have a slight fever in the early stages and to lose weight.

Aches and Pains

The first symptoms of arthritis are often just generalized aches and pains, very similar in fact to those that develop during flu, but the difference is that they last much longer. Stiffness of the hands and the other joints is a common feature. This is particularly noticeable first thing in the morning and it may take several hours before the disabling effects of the stiffness subside. At this stage, sufferers complain more of this than of pain.

Arthritis

Later with the further development of arthritis, the joints become swollen and painful; when pressed upon, they feel tender, and an attempt to use them generates pain. Because of this, the sufferer tries to avoid using the affected joints, with the danger that movement becomes more and more restricted.

Which Joints?

There are certain joints that are especially prone to be affected by rheumatoid arthritis. These are the finger joints (particularly those at the bases and in the middle of the fingers but not those toward the fingertips), the wrist joints, the knees, and those at the bases of the toes. But, in fact, it is possible for any of

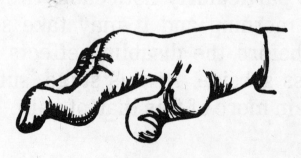

the joints in the body that contain this particular lining tissue (called synovial membrane) — such as the ankles, elbows, shoulders, and hips — to be involved, but these other joints are affected less frequently.

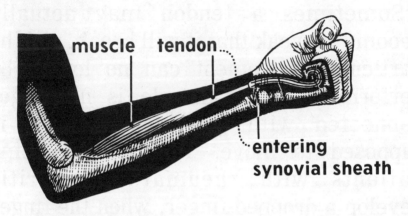

muscle tendon

entering synovial sheath

And Tendons?

The muscles supply the forces that operate the joints by means of their leaders or tendons; these tendons are attached to the bones so that when muscles contract joints move. Because some of the tendons themselves run through sliding tunnels which are lined by a sheath of the same type of synovial membrane as the joints, they also can be affected.

113

This sheath may become so inflamed that scar tissue forms between the tendon and its tunnel. Consequently, the tendon movements become stiff, or the underlying tendon may be "eaten" by this inflamed synovial membrane.

Sometimes a tendon may actually become so weak that it will break, and the particular movement can no longer be performed — the muscle is no longer connected with the bone that it is supposed to move. This is why some patients with rheumatoid arthritis develop a dropped finger, when the finger

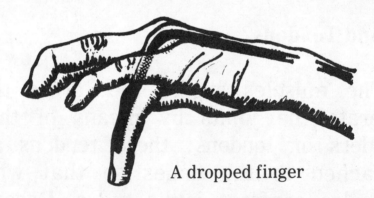

A dropped finger

can grip but can no longer be straightened, due to a torn tendon at the back of the wrist.

Finally, a tendon may get displaced. When this happens, any attempt to move the joint increases the deformity.

What Happens in Severe Arthritis?

Certain characteristic deformities develop in someone with severe arthritis — you may perhaps have noticed them, for they usually involve the hands. The fingers may bend over sideways and no longer remain in line with the forearm; or the finger joints themselves may become bent in various strange directions, so that it becomes difficult to use them. This is partly due to damage to the finger joints,

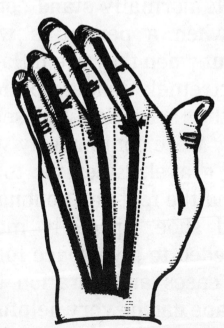

Displacement of the fingers sideways

but more often it reflects the displacement of tendons which pull the bones in the wrong directions.

Another problem is difficulty in bending or straightening the elbow. This may sound rather mundane but it is not. Imagine yourself finding it difficult to eat because you cannot put your hand to your mouth, or — even more frustrating — imagine not being able to scratch the back of your neck or to comb your hair.

Another exasperating problem is the severe involvement of the joints at the base of the toes — as frequently happens. These joints normally stand considerable pressure when a person is walking or running. But when they are inflamed, they become extremely tender; patients often describe the sensation as seeming as though they were continuously walking on pebbles or gravel. Later the toes get out of shape and the foot can no longer fit into a standard shoe. Specially made shoes may be needed to give space for the toes. In severe cases an operation to restore the foot shape can be very helpful.

Finally, there is an almost self-imposed

deformity: when the knees are badly affected by arthritis it is possible to obtain some relief when lying in bed by putting a pillow under the knees. This generates a terrible problem, however, for the knees may stiffen in the bent position. The result, of course, is that in addition to the posture being ugly and awkward, it is extremely difficult to walk. It is therefore imperative for patients with arthritis never to lie with pillows under their knees — the immediate relief gained is just not worth the future problems. Special splints are made by the doctor or occupational therapist for the individual patient. These splints enable the patient to rest the joints and prevent the bent-knee deformity.

TREATMENT

A massive research program has been launched in the last few years in an attempt to determine the cause of rheumatoid arthritis. It is essential to discover if there is any infecting organism that might be responsible for the onset of

117

the disease. Once the disease is initiated there is probably some sort of vicious-circle mechanism by which the inflammation becomes self-perpetuating, even when the original cause has long since disappeared. Some of the possible ways in which the mechanism might perpetuate itself are understood, but nothing is completely proved and many more scientific studies are needed. If this circle could be broken in some way, then perhaps the disease could be cured. Indeed, the pace of medical research is such that we can reasonably hope to find the cure for rheumatoid arthritis one day.

But even if we cannot talk of a cure yet, there are several methods of treating this disease that are important as a means of providing relief from pain, preventing unnecessary deformities, and enabling the sufferer to be as independent as possible. Because of the significance of these methods and because the disease is so common, the treatment will be discussed in some detail. They are divided into the following categories:

1. Rest
2. Occupational therapy, aids, appliances, and adaptations in the home
3. Splints and plaster casts
4. Physical therapy
5. Drugs
6. Surgery

The Importance of Rest

There is no doubt that periods of rest are of the greatest value to patients with rheumatoid arthritis. When the disease is really active and severe, then complete bed rest is essential. People are often admitted to a hospital for this reason alone. It is virtually impossible for some to obtain complete rest at home, as most young housewives with small children would agree.

Psychological factors are also important. Mental rest is equally as important as physical rest; being separated from the problems arising at home is just as valuable as the physical rest.

Confined to bed At this particular stage, apart from getting up to go to the bathroom or to wash, the patient is confined to bed. And this does not just mean lazily lying in bed all day. The position of the body in bed is important: the bed itself should be firm — with no sagging in the middle. The patient should lie flat and sleep with one pillow and, to repeat an important earlier warning, pillows beneath the knees are emphatically forbidden. That may sound like a lot of regulations for just lying in bed, but there are still more to come. If possible, a board should be provided at the foot of the bed for the feet to press on, so as to keep the ankles at right angles to the body, thus preventing them from becoming bent pointing downward. The pressure of bedclothes on painful feet can create trouble and so a cradle over the feet, under the bedclothes, is often used. If this is not available at home, a large cardboard box with two adjacent sides removed is just as protective, although perhaps not as sophisticated. Finally, when the patient sits up in bed, the back of the neck should be properly supported by pillows.

Taking it easy The period for complete bed rest for people with severe disease need only be two or three weeks. But anyone suffering from rheumatoid arthritis should take a series of rests throughout the day.

Try to spend at least an hour extra in bed each night. Get up late, put your feet up for an hour after lunch, and go to bed early. Avoid social commitments that would keep you out late at night.

One of the best ways of starting the day for a rheumatoid arthritis sufferer is, as for anyone else, with a cup of coffee, but this should be brought at least an hour before the patient is due to rise and should be used to help swallow the first pain-relieving tablets of the day. By the time the patient gets up, the pills will have begun to work. A warm bath immediately after rising will ease much of the morning stiffness, leaving the joints in reasonable working order.

A word of caution is needed here. With

early rheumatoid arthritis, rest is helpful, often immediately and obviously so. With "burnt out" rheumatoid arthritis of some years' duration rest can be overdone — the joints, though out of shape, need to be used and the muscles need to be kept in training, just as in a person without arthritis. In the intermediate stages between early and "burnt out" disease, it is often a matter of trial and error to see just how much rest and how much exercise are beneficial, and the guidance of the doctor or physical therapist should be followed.

Remember also that the stiffness that comes on in the morning or after resting is not caused by resting alone, and attempts should not be made to work it off by vigorous exercise. Rather, it reflects the exercise of the previous day. So do not be afraid of extra rest periods. A short rest after lunch can be the determining factor as to whether the sufferer can cope with the afternoon or not.

Others need to understand the predicament of the sufferer and help when possible. This is particularly important for the patient who is both a housewife and mother; it should be understood by her family that she is no longer able to cope with much of the physical work involved in running the house. Other members of the family must help her with the shopping, the domestic chores, and the younger children. Such help will lighten her burden considerably.

Occupational Therapy, Aids, Appliances, and Adaptations in the Home

It is easy — but not practical — to believe that life can continue in the same way for sufferers as it did before the onset of the disease. That is not to say that rheumatoid arthritis should be seen as a crisis or a disaster, but it should be recognized as a *real* situation that needs to be coped with through certain adaptations. The whole organization of the patient's daily life must be rethought. Living conditions can be designed to make life much easier for the sufferer. The occupational therapist from the hospital has received special training in this field, so it may help patients with arthritis to go and chat with her about their own particular problems. The occupational therapist may well want to visit the home with the patient to actually see what difficulties may be encountered, before she makes useful and helpful suggestions.

The kitchen, for example, is often poorly designed, forcing the poor housewife to walk many unnecessary miles during the day while carrying saucepans between the sink and the stove, and food between work surfaces and the refrigerator. Simple rearrangement of the kitchen can help her considerably. For instance, the stove should be next to a working surface and near the sink, so that the housewife, if she has a heavy saucepan to empty, can slide it straight across from the stove without having to lift it physically.

There is a wide variety of specially designed cooking utensils for patients with arthritic problems. For instance, if the patient has a problem holding an ordinary knife because her fingers will not bend sufficiently to grip, then a knife with a specially thick handle may be the answer.

The toilet can also be a problem. Patients with severe hip or knee diseases may have difficulty in getting on and off it. A simple grab rail and an adaptation of the bowl to give it a high seat may improve the situation. Another exasperating factor is that quite often the bathroom is virtually inaccessible, being up one or two flights of stairs which the patient finds impossible to climb. Today there are several models of completely hygienic and aesthetically acceptable chemical commodes, which can be wheeled to the patient and then stored away without any unpleasantness. A severely crippled patient may have great difficulty with personal hygiene after using the toilet. For them a bidet with a spray followed by warm air for drying can be supplied. A specially designed seat can be used if the patient has difficulty climbing in or out of the bath.

Even turning a door knob can be very difficult for a person with a weak hand. The most sensible suggestion is that these be replaced by lever-type door handles.

Combs with long handles, gadgets for turning difficult faucets, and devices for putting on and taking off stockings are all readily available. There is a wide range of aids and appliances for disabled people. If a disabled person has a problem, someone has almost certainly invented an answer to it.

People with deformed feet have enormous difficulty in getting comfortable footwear. Suitable shoes cannot be found in ordinary shoe shops, and it is becoming increasingly difficult and expensive to have shoes made. Not having a shoe that fits the foot means essentially that it is impossible to go out of doors. There is now, however, a technique for taking plaster-of-Paris impressions of the feet and sending these impressions to a shoe factory that makes the shoes accordingly.

A patient who has difficulty in getting around may also be helped by the simple method of using a cane or, in more severe disease, by the use of crutches or a walker.

For many people these special aids, appliances, and adaptations of the home do, in fact, represent the dividing line between dependence on others and independent living. As such, their importance must not be underestimated — they are just as important to arthritics as glasses are to the shortsighted.

Splints and Plaster Casts

Just comfortably supporting an inflamed joint may provide a lot of relief from pain. In the early stages of rheumatoid arthritis in those few patients in whom the process is very severe, the doctor will often prescribe that the joint be placed in a plaster-of-Paris splint. This applies particularly to the wrist, knee, and ankle joints.

If the knee is badly damaged, problems may arise when the patient starts to walk again. A much stronger splint, perhaps made out of plastic, is then used to support the knee, enabling the patient to walk without the joint undergoing strain until the muscles have recovered enough to hold the joint normally.

Physical Therapy

The purpose of physical therapy is to maintain and improve the range of the movements of the joints and to increase the strength of the muscles that control them. Various exercises should be performed with these aims in mind.

Exercise In the acute stages of the disease it is best to stay immobilized and probably even to have the acutely inflamed joints placed in splints. When the acute inflammation subsides, the physical therapist will start very gentle exercises to regain the range of movement. Later, exercises will be more active and directed to regaining strength in the muscles. These exercises will be individually designed for the patient by the physician or physical therapist, who will gradually increase the number of times the patient is to repeat them.

The following exercises are examples of ones that might be suggested after there is no evidence of acute inflammation.

For the wrist, bending the wrist back while making a gentle fist and then bending it down and straightening the fingers can be helpful.

Similarly, the elbow should be bent and then straightened several times.

The shoulders can be moved in a complete circle. The patient stands or sits upright and moves one shoulder at a time in all directions. If this is too painful, a similar exercise can be done lying on a bed. Gravity then assists and it is easier to stretch the shoulder fully by reaching through the bars at the head of the bed.

A wide range of movements in the hip and ankle joints should also be practiced.

Knee exercises are most important; the quadriceps muscle — that is the large muscle lying in front of the thigh — tends to waste away very rapidly when there is disease in the knee. It is possible to prevent this to a considerable extent if the quadriceps muscle is exercised. The patient lies flat in bed and forcibly pushes the back of the knee downward onto the bed, at the same time contracting the

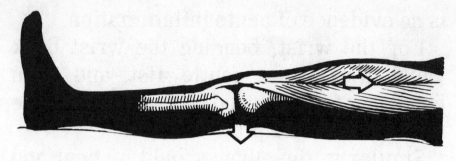
Quadriceps muscle

muscle and pulling up the kneecap. Another exercise is to lie flat in bed, tighten up the kneecap, and then raise the whole leg, keeping the knee as straight as possible. As the strength of the muscle improves, this exercise can be made harder by adding weights to the ankle. The suggested way of doing this is to hang a bag with cans of soup over the ankle, or special ankle weights may be bought. The straight leg is elevated to a forty-five-degree angle, held for five seconds, then lowered again.

The principle behind using weights in exercising is to increase the amount of resistance being given to the muscle. The decision about increasing the weights is made by the physician or physical therapist, who will also instruct the patient about the number of times he should do the exercises during the day.

The importance of exercise when the patient is recovering from a flare-up of the disease cannot be overestimated. Joints and muscles that are not exercised do not do as well as those that are. Exercise is one of the most important means of avoiding deformity. The exercises, however, must be selected and taught by a person trained to do so.

Hydrotherapy One way of coping with the problem of weight is with the use of water. Physical therapy exercises in water are therefore often prescribed. This is part of what is termed hydrotherapy. Basically, these exercises are performed in a large, shallow, warm swimming pool. There is usually a slope on one side of the pool so that patients can walk down to the required depth. Once in the pool, the weight of the patient's body is considerably less (because it is supported by the water), so that the painful joint can be moved with much less effort. It is then very easy to do hip and other exercises.

Of all the methods of getting stiff joints working again, hydrotherapy in a warm swimming pool is the most pleasant and effective. In the past the great spas and watering places of Europe built up their reputations partly on the results of treatment in swimming baths fed by natural hot springs. Spas and spa therapy are dealt with in more detail in Chapter 12.

Hydrotherapy, although beneficial in all except the early stages of rheumatoid arthritis, is also very tiring and should always be followed by a period of rest, with the patient wrapped in a large, warm towel. If hydrotherapy is prescribed for the morning, then nothing active should be planned for the afternoon or evening of that day.

Rheumatoid arthritis patients can often help themselves by performing these exercises in their own bathtub or in a public swimming pool if the water is not cold. And if that seems too conspicuous, they can simply swim, which is a very good exercise in itself.

Heat And if swimming seems an appealing type of therapy, heat for the less active must surely sound even more attractive and comforting. Relief for a painful joint can often be obtained at home by applying moist heat. This may be done by heating a silica-gel hot pack in hot water and placing it over thick turkish toweling, then covering the joint for the twenty or so minutes it takes the pack to cool down.

A hot pack cannot bring heat to all sides of the joints of the fingers, however, and therefore another method of applying heat is used for the painful hand. This is the wax bath. A special grade of paraffin wax is used for this purpose and can be bought from the druggist. It is essential to use the right wax, as other waxes melt at too high a temperature, which would mean that if the hand was dipped into them, the skin would be severely burned. When used at home, this wax should never be melted directly on an electric or gas stove, for it can easily catch fire. It should be melted in a double boiler so that it is gently steamed from beneath, and only heated to the temperature that is required to melt it. It is allowed to cool until a skin forms on the top. The hand is dipped in and out of the wax about half a dozen times until it has a thick coating of warm wax around it. Then it is placed in a plastic bag wrapped in a towel to preserve the heat. This will provide gentle heat in the inflamed area for about half an hour or more. At the end of this time the wax glove can be stripped off and returned for remelting. If exercises have been prescribed for the hands, now is the time to do them, when the hands are warm and relaxed.

In addition to wax baths, there is a variety of complex electrical apparatus which are used in hospitals for applying heat, but they are not practical for the home as they must be used under the supervision of a trained physical therapist.

Medical Control of Rheumatoid Arthritis

The drugs used can be considered under six headings:
1. Drugs that relieve pain and suppress inflammation
2. Drugs that produce remissions of rheumatoid arthritis
3. Steroid and cortisone preparations
4. Drugs that suppress immunity
5. Drugs that help deal with complications of rheumatoid arthritis, such as anemia
6. New drugs for the treatment of rheumatoid arthritis

Drugs that relieve pain and inflammation We are all familiar with aspirin as a drug for relieving pain — and as such it is the most useful drug for treating rheumatoid arthritis. However, patients must consult their doctor, agree on an appropriate dosage, and then stick to it. If taken in the full dosage, it will actually suppress the inflammation; this has been proved by a very clever study in which the sizes of inflamed finger joints were measured using jewelers' rings.

But every medicament known to physicians can produce undesirable side effects. Aspirin is no exception, although on the whole it is a fairly safe drug. Many tons of aspirin are consumed every year in this country and yet the frequency of side effects remains very low.

One of the possible problems with aspirin is that it is liable to produce indigestion and stomach pains. If they develop, the doctor must be consulted for advise as to whether the drug should be stopped. There are some specially prepared formulations and derivatives of aspirin available. Some of these have a protective coating that helps to prevent the aspirin from irritating the stomach lining.

Another disadvantage of aspirin is the number of tablets that have to be taken — sometimes twelve or more a day. There is now a liquid form of aspirin that is taken only two or three times a day for the same effect.

Alternative available drugs that

similarly reduce pain and suppress inflammation are indomethacin (Indocin®), phenylbutazone (Butazolidin®), and many others. Indomethacin causes headaches in some people and can occasionally produce the same sort of indigestion problems as aspirin. Phenylbutazone may sometimes produce stomach ulcers and, rarely, disturbances in the blood that can be serious. Any patients taking these drugs should be reviewed regularly by their doctors.

Phenacetin must be mentioned here in terms of a warning. This is a drug that is particularly effective in relieving pain, but unfortunately if it is taken for many years, it can lead to severe kidney damage. It should be completely avoided by patients with arthritis, some of whom need to take tablets daily for many years. Phenacetin is not usually sold as an isolated drug but it is often present as one of a mixture of compounds presented under various trade names at the druggist's. The commonest of these contain aspirin, phenacetin, and caffein and are used for headaches. Any arthritic must ask the pharmacist or else read the small print on the container to make sure that no phenacetin is present in the tablets that he is purchasing.

Drugs that produce remissions of rheumatoid arthritis There are certain drugs that function, not to relieve pain and inflammation in the same way as aspirin, but to encourage a remission — or a clearing up — of the disease two or three months after the start of the treatment. They are the nearest thing that medicine has to a cure of the disease. Unfortunately, they do not work in all cases, nor can the benefit be guaranteed to last. They are usually given with aspirin or other pain-relievers.

These drugs that produce remissions were discovered to be useful purely by accident.

In the days before the new antibiotics became available for treating tuberculosis, gold injections were often used for that disease. They did not have much effect on tuberculosis, but it was observed that when some patients with

138

rheumatoid arthritis were treated (because at one time this disease was mistakenly thought to be related to tuberculosis), the arthritis improved. Similarly, it was found that some of the drugs used in the prevention of malaria in people going to the tropics also led to considerable improvement in arthritis patients. For these reasons, the use of these two types of drugs has been carefully tried out in patients with rheumatoid arthritis — and has proved to be beneficial.

But that is where the good luck stopped. Although gold is effective, there are undesirable side effects, particularly involving the skin, the kidneys, and the blood. If the patient develops itching or any sort of rash, then it is essential that he tell the doctor and that the gold injections be stopped. Because of this element of doubt, precautions are always taken: the urine is tested before each injection, the patient is given regular blood counts, and if he develops a sore throat or other ill effects, then the gold is discontinued. Despite all this, gold remains one of the most effective treatments we have and, with strict precautions, should be safe.

The drugs discovered from treating malaria, chloroquine (Aralen®) and hydroxychloroquine (Plaquenil®), also have their own unwanted effects. One of these relates to retinal damage to the eyes; it is absolutely essential that the eyes of patients taking these drugs be checked by an eye specialist every six to twelve months. In a recent review one American hospital found that serious eye trouble caused by these drugs occurred only once in 7,000 patients — so it is not common.

One of the most recent developments is another drug, called penicillamine, which should be mentioned here. It is related to penicillin but it is not itself an antibiotic. It is made by the chemical breakdown of penicillin — a wasteful process, as it takes fifty or more doses of penicillin to make one dose of penicillamine. Not surprisingly, penicillamine has been very expensive, but new, wholly synthetic chemical methods are expected to bring the price down. The history of penicillamine is interesting, since it was first discovered by Dr. (now Professor Sir) Ernst Chain at Oxford, the man who did most to rediscover Fleming's original, unexploited findings and to develop penicillin as a practical and lifesaving antibiotic

Among many other advances, penicillin, as well as helping thousands of soldiers with infected war wounds, was able to destroy the micro-organism called hemolytic streptococcus, the direct cause of "strep throat" and the indirect cause of rheumatic fever, a disease that has now virtually disappeared from affluent countries (see Chapter 9). Chain's other research, in discovering penicillamine, did not have the same immediate dramatic effect on rheumatoid arthritis as did the discovery of penicillin on rheumatic fever. It was nearly thirty years before the possible benefits were widely appreciated, because the benefits, when they do occur, are delayed and undramatic in their appearance.

Penicillamine is a relatively simple

drug, but it has numerous interesting properties and has now been used continuously for over fifteen years in certain rare inherited "chemical" diseases. Because of this, a lot is known about the problems and benefits of its long-term use. Its use in rheumatoid arthritis dates from about 1968. It was observed that it could break down the large, abnormal protein molecules called rheumatoid factor, which circulate in the blood of most sufferers and which are the basis of the blood test for rheumatoid arthritis. Penicillamine could turn the test from positive to negative, though to most observers it did not seem to improve the patient's condition. But one or two persistent and perceptive doctors, in particular a New York physician named Jaffe, realized that improvement might be long delayed. Jaffe continued to use this drug, which others had thought too expensive and ineffective. Since he did not do a modern, carefully controlled clinical trial, his ideas were not generally accepted until such trials were done in the early 1970s in Britain.

Penicillamine is not an easy drug to handle. Not everyone can take it. "Go low, go slow" is the motto for treatment; the dosage given is very low at first and then very, very cautiously increased. Given medical supervision and the use of precautions very like those needed for gold injections, treatment has proved to be of great benefit for many sufferers.

Cortisone and other steroids These drugs could properly be included with aspirin and the others that suppress inflammation and relieve pain, but for emphasis and convenience they are discussed separately. They have a dramatic — indeed, almost miraculous — effect in relieving arthritis. Once a patient with rheumatoid arthritis starts taking either cortisone or its derivatives (prednisone, prednisolone, and similar steroid compounds), all the symptoms and signs of arthritis can disappear virtually overnight. The introduction of these drugs was accompanied, not surprisingly, by an enthusiastic belief that here at last was a cure of rheumatoid arthritis.

But, sadly, these hopes have not been sustained; the drugs are certainly very effective on a short-term basis, but in the long run, patients generally do as well or better without them. Moreover, they can also produce very severe side effects. The principal problems of these particular drugs are that they are likely to produce indigestion or stomach ulcers, and that they can seriously weaken the bones and muscles. Also, if large doses are used, after a few months of treatment the face becomes red and rounded (moon face), and women may grow facial hair. Doctors therefore try to avoid their use whenever possible.

But sometimes it is not possible. Steroids are so effective that in severe disease their immediate use may be required: nothing else will help. However, the dose is reduced as soon as possible and restricted to the essential minimum. From time to time, efforts are made to withdraw the drugs entirely. For long-term use, these drugs are relatively safe if taken in very low doses. The temptation to gradually increase the amount must be strictly resisted.

Any patient who is receiving steroid preparations must carry a steroid identity card at all times. This is because dangerous complications may follow if their use is suddenly stopped for any reason. The card contains details of the steroid preparation that the individual is taking — that is, how much and for how long — together with his doctor's name, address, and telephone number. If the patient should be run over by a bus, suffer from a heart attack, need an emergency operation, or if anything else happens that makes him unable to give this information, the card will tell any medical person who is present that steroids are essential.

If the arthritis is generally under good control but one or two joints are inflamed, it is sometimes possible to inject steroids directly into them. This will control those particular joints but is effective only for a few weeks, especially when injections are given into the knee and other weight-bearing joints. In the non-weight-bearing joints, especially those of the fingers, modern derivatives of cortisone may be effective and long-lasting. But these injections require the skills of a specialist.

Drugs that suppress immunity It has recently been found that a special group of drugs will suppress the immunity mentioned at the beginning of this chapter and can be effective in patients with arthritis. However, their use is restricted to patients with very severe disease. Patients must be kept under close observation by a doctor and must have regular and frequent blood checks to make sure that the correct dose is not being exceeded.

Some remarkable improvements have occurred in patients who failed on all other treatments, but these powerful drugs are definitely only indicated in very special circumstances.

Drugs to treat the complications of rheumatoid arthritis Many patients with rheumatoid arthritis are more ill than they need be, not because of the arthritis but because of one of its complications.

Anemia is one of the commonest of these, and it is surprising how frequent it is and how much better patients can cope with their arthritis when the anemia is detected and cured.

Anemia is usually due to iron deficiency and is treated by iron pills or injections. Patients with severe disabilities are also prone to anemia from poor nutrition. They have difficulty in getting food, or, having gotten it, in cooking and preparing it, especially if they live alone. There may then be other dietary deficiencies as well, for which the treatment may of course be different.

Patients with rheumatoid arthritis are prone to low-grade infections, and treatment with the appropriate antibiotic will lead to great improvement.

New drugs for rheumatoid arthritis One fact that has become clear from discussing the drugs used for rheumatoid arthritis is the need for research into new — and old — drugs.

Many new drugs are being developed for the treatment of rheumatoid arthritis. Some of these represent real advances and others only mimic the effects of preparations in current use. Research into drugs is essential. It is imperative to find out precisely how these drugs work. If it is possible to identify the ways in which they produce good effects and to learn how to avoid the harmful effects, then it may be possible to design a successful new drug.

In clinical practice it can be difficult to decide whether a new drug is of real value, especially if it is presented in a brightly colored form. The patients may believe in it and feel that it must be doing them some good, and even the doctor can be misled in a similar way. For this reason, trials of new drugs must be designed carefully and comparisons drawn with drugs of known value, so that the true worth of the preparations can be estimated properly. The long delay in the introduction of penicillamine is an example of what may happen to a useful drug if a modern clinical trial is not done.

Surgical Treatment of Rheumatoid Arthritis

In the last few years rheumatologists have cooperated with orthopedic surgeons to develop a combined approach in treating these patients. Many new operations are being performed and they have dramatically improved the outlook for patients with joint damage.

In the early stages of arthritis, the inflamed synovium or joint lining may be removed by an operation known as synovectomy. Similarly, the sheath of a tendon is lined with synovium and if this is inflamed, then this tissue can also be removed.

Another situation that benefits from surgery is a nerve that is trapped by the inflamed and swollen tissue. A common site for this is at the wrist; here, the nerve passes through the front of the wrist to supply the index, middle, and half the ring finger. The trapped nerve produces "pins and needles" and a feeling of numbness in these fingers. Freeing this nerve by a very minor operation will immediately remove this symptom.

In advanced severe disease there have been some exciting developments in the replacement of damaged joints by artificial joints. The most successful of these operations has been on the hip joint, where it can be expected that over 90 percent of the replaced hips will function successfully. These operations should provide complete relief from pain and a good range of movement. New plastic joints are now being used for the fingers as well and have proved very effective, correcting much of the deformity and allowing a better use of the hands. Replacing the knee is an operation that is still being developed; it can be very successful in some patients but has not yet reached the same stage of perfection as operations on the hip.

THE OUTLOOK FOR RHEUMATOID PATIENTS

After this rather gloomy account, any arthritic readers must surely have been plunged into despair — or put the book away after the first few depressing sentences — and are perhaps anticipating severe crippling in their own particular case.

Nil desperandum! (Do not despair!) The majority of patients with early rheumatoid arthritis have a transient attack which will clear up completely. In many of these patients symptoms are never sufficiently severe to warrant medical attention, and of those that are seen by a general practitioner, only a few are severe enough to require that the patient be seen by an arthritis specialist or be sent to a hospital.

And for those who are sent to a hospital, here are the not-so-grim statistics: they are by far the worst cases, and yet of these patients, in a quarter the disease will clear up completely without any remaining disability. An additional quarter will heal, leaving slight joint damage but not enough to interfere significantly with their working lives. Forty percent will suffer continued disability, which means that they may expect to suffer recurrent pain and be on drugs to control the arthritis, but nevertheless they will not be incapacitated or bedridden. It is only 10 percent or less of these patients who risk becoming severely crippled.

Another factor that also brightens the outlook for patients has already been mentioned at the beginning of this section: a massive research program is at present under way to try to determine the cause of arthritis.

Much research is being done on the mechanisms of immunity and how they become disturbed in rheumatoid arthritis. Other studies are being directed at the actual mechanism by which various types of deformity develop. Many mechanical factors are involved and a better understanding of these will lead to a better approach toward medical and surgical treatment.

5

Diseases Resembling Rheumatoid Arthritis

In writing a book of this nature, there is always the problem that there are a number of less common items that do not readily fall into any of the standard chapters. In order to be comprehensive, a chapter describing these various less common types of inflammatory arthritis and rheumatism is therefore included. Many of these conditions can affect the spine and have already been given a brief mention in Chapter 2.

ARTHRITIS AND PSORIASIS

Psoriasis is a curious but very common condition of the skin which is related to certain forms of arthritis. Once seen psoriasis is easily recognized — it appears as patches of thickened red skin that have a strong tendency to flake. Commonly sited on the back of the elbow, the front of the knee, and in the scalp, psoriasis can also appear anywhere on the trunk or limbs. As with so many medical conditions, the precise cause of this disease is a mystery. Studies of the skin itself, including parts of the skin not affected by the actual rash, have shown that there are significant abnormalities in the behavior of the skin cells and also of the smallest capillary blood vessels that bring oxygen and other nutrients to the skin.

Psoriasis can start at any age and often begins in childhood. It occurs in several members of a family more often than would be expected by chance, so perhaps there is some inherited predisposition to it. Sometimes one meets families in which one member has psoriasis and another member has mild arthritis and yet another member has both. But the true nature of this inheritance — if that is what it is — is still unknown.

Rheumatoid Arthritis Coinciding with Psoriasis

Confusion may arise because both rheumatoid arthritis and psoriasis are common conditions, so that by sheer coincidence alone they occasionally develop together. The arthritic problem is exactly the same as in any other patient with rheumatoid arthritis (as described in Chapter 4).

Psoriatic Arthropathy

Rheumatoid arthritis coinciding with psoriasis should not, however, be confused with the type of arthritis directly associated with psoriasis — so-called psoriatic arthropathy. Despite certain superficial resemblances to rheumatoid arthritis, this condition is an entirely separate disease with important distinguishing features.

Psoriatic arthropathy can affect any joint, but in contrast to rheumatoid arthritis it often affects only one or two joints. The joint becomes inflamed, causing pain and swelling which then limits movement. The joints near the tips of the finger (which are hardly ever affected in rheumatoid arthritis) are especially prone to inflammation. When these joints are inflamed, the corresponding fingernails also show direct damage due to psoriasis. In its mildest form there is very tiny pitting spread randomly over the nail, which is only detected on very close examination, but later the nail becomes severely damaged and is seen to be thick and discolored. The nail may even become partly separated from the tip of the finger by a thick white chalky material.

Psoriatic arthropathy can sometimes severely damage a joint and the inflammatory process may eat away the bony surfaces. In general, however, the arthritis of psoriatic arthropathy is less severe than ordinary rheumatoid arthritis and patients do better in the long run.

Psoriasis and the Spine

Involvement of the spine is another —
but uncommon — type of arthritis
associated with psoriasis. In its simplest
form there is inflammation at the bottom
of the spine around the sacroiliac joints.
These, you may remember, are the same
joints that are involved in ankylosing
spondylitis, and spinal changes that are
similar to ankylosing spondylitis may
develop with psoriasis. The low back
pain and stiffness that characterize
inflammation of the sacroiliac joints are
the first symptoms, but the arthritis may
spread from these joints up the spine
toward the neck. After the initial stages in
inflammation the bony changes of
ankylosing spondylitis may develop with
similar results — back pain and back
stiffness, sometimes to the point of
rigidity. It can be impossible to
distinguish psoriatic involvement of the
spine from ankylosing spondylitis.

Psoriasis and Gout

Finally a brief reference must be made to the fact that the abnormal biochemical changes in the skin may lead to excessive production of uric acid in the blood which consequently may produce gout. This is rare, but when it occurs, it leads to great confusion in deciding upon the cause of arthritis.

REITER'S SYNDROME

The tradition of naming places after the explorers who discovered them seems to have seeped into medical custom, where several names of diseases have been derived from the first ostensible discoverer of the condition. Hans Reiter in 1916 described the case of a Prussian cavalry officer serving in the Balkans who developed acute arthritis together with inflammation of the eyes and a discharge from the penis. Since then, the disease has been called Reiter's disease or Reiter's syndrome, but in fact the true credit belongs to an Englishman — Sir Benjamin

Brodie — who described the disease almost a hundred years earlier, in 1818.

A Type of VD?

It has been suggested that there is a possible relationship between Reiter's syndrome and venereal disease. Many cases occur as a form of venereal disease, but not all. Reiter's syndrome may also follow as a result of infective diarrhea.

The disease is probably due to some sort of virus and is transmitted directly from one person to another. Outbreaks of Reiter's syndrome have been described aboard ships in circumstances suggesting this type of infection. It is far more common in men than women and most frequent in young adults, although it may persist and indeed appear in older people. The disease occurs in those who have frequent sexual intercourse with many different partners. However, direct proof is still lacking, and there are probably additional factors that predispose certain individuals to develop this disease.

The Symptoms

The early symptoms of Reiter's syndrome are certainly suggestive of venereal disease, usually including a slight discharge from the penis. Within a couple of weeks, an inflammation called conjunctivitis develops in one or both eyes, and shortly after this, arthritis appears. The joints, often those of the feet and knees but sometimes elsewhere, become swollen and very painful. Ulcers may appear, usually on the penis or inside the mouth. Finally, there also may be a skin rash (which can resemble some varieties of psoriasis) that appears on the soles of the feet and then perhaps on the rest of the body. As this description implies, Reiter's syndrome can be a very unpleasant disease.

Treatment

Treatment includes antibiotics, antiinflammatory drugs, physical therapy, and rest; given these, the condition usually settles down within a few weeks or months. Sometimes the disease may reappear, but such recurrences subside also. Occasionally the feet may become badly affected, and changes in the spine, similar to those of ankylosing spondylitis, may develop. But fortunately, the great majority of cases recover completely.

ULCERATIVE COLITIS AND REGIONAL ENTERITIS

Ulcerative colitis and regional enteritis are both conditions in which there is inflammation of the bowel, and both are diseases that sometimes have the additional affliction of being accompanied by forms of arthritis.

The two conditions, however, do differ in many details from each other. To understand these differences, a point of clarification is perhaps needed: in its passage through the body, food which enters the stomach passes out through the duodenum into the small intestine and then into the large intestine before any waste materials are lost. Ulcerative colitis is characterized by persistent

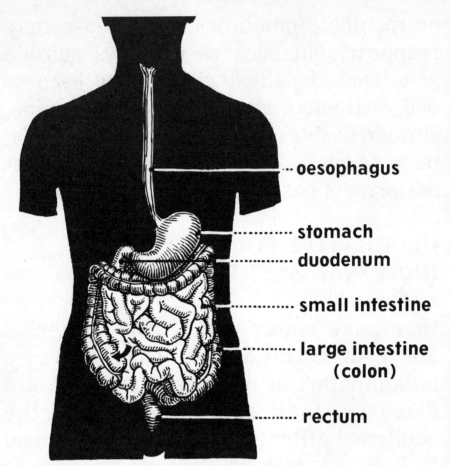

The digestive tract

inflammation of the large intestine, producing recurrent and sometimes severe diarrhea. Regional enteritis, on the other hand, more frequently involves the small intestine.

Similar types of arthritis may complicate both conditions. Inflammatory arthritis may occur in either the limbs or the spine.

Arthritis in the Limbs

The more common complication with ulcerative colitis and regional enteritis is arthritis of the limbs. This is usually in the knees but can sometimes also affect the feet or elsewhere. Again, it is the same story — the joints become swollen, inflamed, and painful, and may be difficult to move. Fortunately, the arthritis is usually mild and clears up spontaneously within a few weeks, rarely leaving behind any permanent damage. Usually, the degree of inflammation of the joints corresponds to that in the intestine, so that when the bowel inflammation improves with treatment, inflammation in the joints subsides.

Arthritis in the Spine

Inflammation of the joints in the spine can also accompany these conditions, but this produces an entirely different form of rheumatism. Again, the sacroiliac joints at the lower end of the spine are affected first, with symptoms that are similar to those of ankylosing spondylitis; pain and stiffness in the low back are increased by resting and are especially bad during the night, while relief is gained through exercise. When the arthritis becomes more severe, inflammation spreads up the spine, revealing itself to be ankylosing spondylitis. The symptoms are precisely the same as described in Chapter 2 — stiffness of the whole spine is present and all movements become very limited. Eventually, the vertebrae can become joined by bone, so that all hope of further movement becomes lost.

Treatment lies in control of the bowel disease and prevention of stiffness by exercises and activity. Drugs such as aspirin or indomethacin are used to damp down inflammation in the joints.

These forms of arthritis are of research interest because they support one theory as to the cause of ankylosing spondylitis. The theory is that some form of infection in the pelvis leads to chronic inflammation of the spine — but only in those people who have an inherited susceptibility. The nature of this inherited predisposition became more clear recently with the simultaneous discovery in Los Angeles and London that nine out of ten people with ankylosing spondylitis belonged to the same white blood cell group, HL-A27 (see page 46).

SYSTEMIC LUPUS ERYTHEMATOSUS AND OTHER AUTOIMMUNE DISEASES

Immunity

There is a custom among many parents to encourage their children to catch certain infections, such as German measles. This is of course no wild desire to nurse their child through these rather irritating conditions, but rather an insurance against their contracting such diseases in future years. In other words, immunity to these particular conditions is encouraged because once a child has had German measles (or chickenpox, mumps, measles, and a host of other infections), he never gets it again. Furthermore, the disease in a child is less severe than in an adult.

The principles of immunization are quite simple although the details are extremely complicated. During the initial infection special proteins called antibodies are produced by the tissues. These antibodies are directed at the particular invading organisms and eventually destroy them. Even after the disease has been wiped out, the antibodies persist in the blood and therefore prevent further attacks. These antibodies can also be stimulated artificially in the body by appropriate injections so as to avoid an attack of a particular disease — as no doubt those of us who travel aboard are aware, for these are the processes of vaccination and immunization that are used for diphtheria, smallpox, measles, yellow fever, typhoid, and countless other diseases.

Autoimmunity

Antibodies therefore have a very important function in the body. They are there to protect us from infections. But occasionally things go wrong. Instead of antibodies being produced to fight against invading bacteria or viruses they are developed against the body's own tissue. When this happens, it is called autoimmunity.

Inflammation due to autoimmunity may occur in many structures in the body, including the joints, lungs, skin, heart, blood cells, kidneys, and so on. This condition — when autoimmunity occurs attacking many parts of the body — is called by the rather complicated name systemic lupus erythematosus.

Systemic Lupus Erythematosus

An analysis of the meaning of this name partly explains the characteristics of the disease:

systemic — spread throughout the entire body

lupus — from the Latin for "wolf," which described the rash that may appear on the face. (It used to be thought to be similar to the effects of a wolf bite.)

erythematosus — from "erythema"

or redness, meaning inflammation occurring in the skin

Systemic lupus erythematosus is obviously a very complicated and unpleasant condition although, fortunately, modern drugs have done much to control it. It is included in this book because a prominent feature of the disease can be inflammation of the joints and rheumatism. Young women are most frequently affected and occasionally it follows the use of certain medicaments.

Related Disorders

There is a variety of related disorders (with equally fascinating names), two of which should be mentioned briefly.

In polyarteritis nodosa there is inflammation of the blood vessels. This may occur in many parts of the body but in particular may affect the blood vessels near joints and produce forms of arthritis.

Scleroderma is a peculiar condition in which there is considerable thickening of the skin. This is most marked in the hands, but may sometimes spread over other parts of the body. Because of this thickening, movement of the limbs, particularly of the hands, becomes very stiff and difficult.

Our understanding of this group of disorders is still limited. Research aimed at investigating the mechanisms of immunity and the disturbances in all these different forms of autoimmune disease is currently being carried out. Rheumatoid arthritis itself is closely related to this group of conditions, and a fuller understanding of one should aid in the understanding of all the others.

VENEREAL DISEASE AND ARTHRITIS

Reiter's syndrome has already been described as one form of venereal disease leading to joint disorders. It was presented earlier in the chapter because of its similarities to the arthritis related to psoriasis and because Reiter's syndrome is not exclusively a result of venereal disease. Many cases follow dysentery.

Venereal diseases can cause a lot of

trouble, but the only ones with which we are concerned in this book are those that are accompanied by forms of arthritis.

Gonorrhea

Gonorrhea is the commonest form of venereal disease in affluent countries, and with the current relaxing of sexual mores, it has become the most prevalent reportable infectious disease in the United States. By 1971, the number of *reported* cases had reached an all-time high figure of 285.2 per 100,000 people — a figure considered to be only the visible tip of the iceberg. It is caused by a tiny rounded organism called the gonococcus, which is transmitted by sexual contact and infects the sexual organs. The major problem with gonorrhea is that although the symptoms in men are obvious and painful, women who are affected often do not know it, so they fail to obtain proper medical treatment and continue to transmit the disease to their partners without ever realizing that they have it.

The onset of gonorrhea is experienced

as a burning pain while passing urine, usually with a discharge from the penis in men. A week or two later the sufferer may become generally ill with aches and pain in many joints due to a generalized infection of the body. Then eventually the infection may focus around one particular joint which becomes acutely inflamed.

Fortunately gonorrhea usually responds successfully to penicillin, but it is most important that this treatment is started as quickly as possible.

Syphilis

Syphilis is a much more serious disease which, although showing an overall decline in the number of reported cases from a peak of 75.6 per 100,000 people in 1947 to 11.5 in 1971, also has been on the increase recently. It is caused by a corkscrew-shaped organism different from the one described above and in time can produce terrible complications in many of the body tissues.

Many years after infection it can damage the nerves in the spinal cord that send the messages of pain from the legs to the brain. This has important results. With this loss of feeling of pain in the legs, the joints can be badly sprained without the person concerned being aware of any trouble at all. Normally, the pain from, say, a sprained ankle stops the sufferer from using it. It hurts too much and he has to rest it, and with rest the damage rapidly heals. However, when pain is absent, continual use of damaged and weakened joints may produce further damage, and this is precisely what may happen in people who have had syphilis. Their joints suffer recurrent damage and eventually become destroyed. Although pain-free, the joints are unstable and easily give way, thus preventing proper use of the limb. This condition occurs most frequently in the feet or knees which are then known as Charcot joints, after a famous French physician who was interested in diseases of nerves.

These painless but damaged Charcot joints are not exclusive to syphilis — they are occasionally found in severe diabetes and in other diseases of the nerves. They sometimes develop (fortunately rarely in the United States) in patients with leprosy when the nerves are damaged by the leprosy bacillus.

6

Ageing, Wear and Tear, and Osteoarthritis

The last two chapters have concentrated on inflammatory types of arthritis; if, however, the doctor finds no evidence of inflammation in the bones and joints then the trouble is quite likely to be due to wear and tear. This process of wearing out of joints has already been described fully in Chapter 1 in relation to the back (lumbar spondylosis) and in Chapter 3 in relation to the neck (cervical spondylosis).

A similar process of wearing out can occur in other joints where it is then called osteoarthrosis or osteoarthritis. Although osteoarthritis can affect many joints at the same time, it should not be regarded as a disease of the entire body like measles or rheumatoid arthritis.

174

Each individual joint must be considered as an isolated problem.

AGEING, OR WEAR AND TEAR

Osteoarthritis is a process that is inextricably related to the ageing of joints. It would be pleasant to believe that we are the same people throughout our lives, but the truth is that we are not. The supple young man of nineteen becomes the stiff old man of ninety with gray hair and a changed face. Similarly, changes also occur in the joints, bones, muscles, and tendons — all the things that can give rise to the various forms of rheumatism.

Most of these changes are painless: the fact that they happen so gradually tends to make them acceptable. It is only when the wearing process starts unusually early, causes pain, or is exaggerated in any way that it is called a disease.

The question that must now be answered is, what exactly happens when the joints age? To understand this process, it is necessary first to comprehend the mechanics by which joints move.

Lubrication and Repair

The human joint has a wonderful system of lubrication. Indeed, engineers would dearly love to be able to reproduce such a remarkable system, and they have in fact learned new principles of engineering by studying the living joint. The natural joint is more slippery than any simple engineering joint or bearing, and only ball bearings and roller bearings create less friction.

How does this system of lubrication work?

1. The two surfaces have a high natural slipperiness. In this they resemble certain plastics that are self-lubricating, i.e., they provide their own lubricant.

2. The surface as revealed under the microscope is not smooth. It is pocketed in a series of minute undulations that trap joint fluid between the two moving parts.

3. The joint fluid is not an oil but a solution of mucus which loses water and

thickens up under pressure.

The surface that forms the slippery end of the bone is called articular cartilage. It grows through childhood, after which it is then formed for life. If it is damaged, it therefore has only a limited power to heal. Partial healing will occur if, for example, a joint has been operated upon and some of the cartilage removed. Or if when a bone breaks the break extends down into the joint, again partial healing will occur.

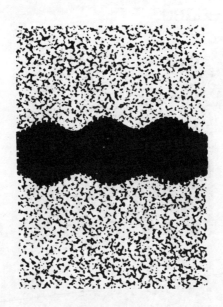

In the moving joint a film of mucus comes between the two surfaces where some of it gets trapped in the little pockets.

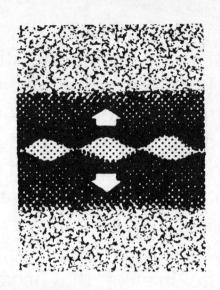

Under pressure the fluid thickens and provides increased lubrication just where it is most needed.

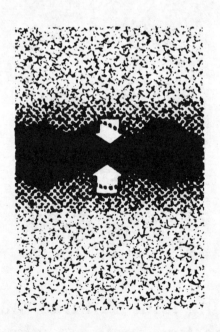

As soon as the pressure is removed from

the surface, water is taken up and the joint fluid resumes its normal thickness.

Failure or Fatigue

Having admired the joint as a remarkable engineering system, the time has now come to question the reasons for its occasional failures or, rather, its less successful functioning.

Articular cartilage, like any other substance, is subject to what the engineers call fatigue. This means that after it has been compressed and released many times, it may pass the limit of its natural resilience and break down.

There are several explanations proffered to account for joints wearing out.

The first theory suggests that joints wear out because of a failure in the lubrication procedures. There is, however, no acceptable evidence of this.

Another theory offered is that the surface is subject to minute abrasive wear which outpaces its replacement.

The third and probably most important

theory has suggested that the breakdown is the result of fatigue due to repeated impact shock. This relates to the bones as well as to the cartilage. The bones in the body have a certain elasticity. In jumping and running they absorb some of the force of the impact, but when old bones stiffen, their elasticity is less and the impact shock on the cartilage is therefore greater. The significance of this theory lies in its practical implications for preventing osteoarthritis. Exponents of such a theory would advise people to avoid being overweight (which increases the force of impact in walking) and to use rubber heels on shoes to cushion the shock of impact, particularly when walking on hard pavements.

Ageing, however, is not the only factor that causes wear and tear. Osteoarthritis is often due to accelerated breakdown. Although most human joints will last in reasonable working order for all of the traditional threescore years and ten — and many even longer — there are certain predisposing factors that encourage early breakdown.

1. The first is incongruity. This means that the two parts of a joint don't fit together as well as they should. Badly made joints of this sort seem to run in certain families. The lack of fit is a frequent cause of trouble in the hip joint. There are also conditions such as congenital dislocation of the hip (when babies are born with the ball of the hip joint out of its socket) and deformities of the joints after operation, which have much the same effect.

2. Sometimes an early joint breakdown can be attributed to chemical or biological changes. The commonest of these is when lime salts are deposited in the cartilage, causing a condition called chondrocalcinosis. This is described in Chapter 7 in more detail. Inflammation damages the joint by eroding some of the surfaces and by damaging the ligaments which are responsible for keeping the joint surfaces in proper alignment. Even if the inflammation gets better, the damage may have been such that the joint is liable to early breakdown later on.

OSTEOARTHRITIS

The Development of Osteoarthritis

The first minute changes of osteoarthritis are visible even in childhood. The surface of the joint begins to break down in one or two places, but the changes are microscopic and because the cartilage is so thick they do not affect the efficiency of the joint. However, by the twenties and thirties the cartilage changes increase so that they can be seen with the naked eye, and they progress until in the forties and fifties the affected joints occasionally begin to feel painful. Each joint responds by attempting to heal itself — sometimes with unfortunate consequences. The new cartilage which grows at the edge of the joint forms a hard knob that later becomes bony. These bone knobs (as you may remember from Chapter 1) are called osteophytes.

These knobby irregularities at the edge of the joint are characteristic features of osteoarthritis. It is the osteophytes which, by obstructing the joint at the hinge, prevent its normal range of movement.

Because each joint must be considered as an isolated problem, it is necessary to look at the way in which osteoarthritis can affect each individual joint. These can be conveniently divided into the non-weight-bearing joints of the arms, and the joints of the legs that take the weight of the body.*

Osteoarthritis in Non-Weight-Bearing Joints

The hands Although many joints in the hand can be affected, there is a tendency for osteoarthritis to appear mainly in the joints at the ends of the fingers and the joint at the base of the thumb. Small knobs, at first soft but later bony, form on the back of these joints.

This produces a characteristic appearance in the finger, and these bony

---

* Wear-and-tear disease of the spine is entirely similar to that in the limb joints. It has already been fully described with reference to the low back and the neck in Chapter 1 and Chapter 3, respectively.

183

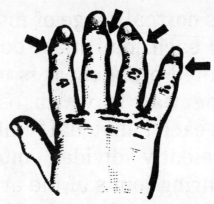

Heberden's nodes

prominences have been called after the physician who first described them. If calling these knobs Heberden's nodes is a form of flattery or praise for William Heberden, then surely he deserved it: by describing this condition in 1803, Heberden stimulated scientific interest in the study of arthritis and rheumatism. As a tribute to his work, an important scientific society for research into arthritis has been named after him.

The pain in the finger when the Heberden's node is forming can be quite annoying and often has a burning quality that is worse at night. But usually the nodes are painless and cause little or no trouble. By contrast, osteoarthritis of the joint at the base of the thumb is more often painful but since there is little to see (the joint is deeper inside the hand), it may not be immediately obvious that it, too, is damaged.

The elbow and shoulder The elbow and shoulder are seldom affected by osteoarthritis. Virtually the only time that they do become involved is after there has been some previous damage. Painful osteoarthritis of the little joint at the top of the shoulder between the collarbone and shoulder blade, is, however, quite frequent, especially as a sporting injury. Surprisingly, the joints of the jaw just in front of the ear can be affected by the same problem and this may, on occasion, make chewing painful.

Osteoarthritis in Weight-Bearing Joints

The knee Osteoarthritis of the knee is very common. The knees creak and may make grating noises, called crepitus, during movement. They become knobby and may be difficult to straighten. The consequences are unfortunate — the subject is liable to be forced into either a bow-legged or knock-kneed position. The latter is more crippling because it is difficult to walk if the knees are continually colliding.

Operations for osteoarthritis of the knee are not as successful as in the hip and so are only performed as a last resort. However, this is a field of medicine where what is difficult today may be commonplace tomorrow.

The feet and ankles The ankles are rarely affected by osteoarthritis. However, the big toe joint, perhaps because of shoe pressure, is prone to the development of a bunion joint, known as hallux valgus. This is really a form of osteoarthritis. Hallux valgus makes shoe-fitting very difficult. Further reference will be made to this in the chapter on feet, Chapter 10.

The hip By far the greatest problem caused by osteoarthritis is the damage and crippling, pain and misery it may cause to the hip. The hip is a fine example

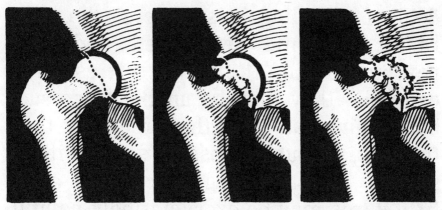

Stages in the development of osteoarthritis of the hip

of a ball-and-socket joint, a joint which enables movement in any direction. But if the hip becomes affected by osteoarthritis it gradually changes in shape as it wears down, into a hinge joint which can only bend backward and forward. Characteristically, these patients cannot part their legs and in women this may make sexual intercourse difficult or impossible by conventional means. Only when the condition becomes really severe does it stop all movement in the joint.

Osteoarthritis of the hip is all too common — indeed it is one of the most frequent reasons why elderly people have to be cared for in nursing homes instead of managing at home. Severe osteoarthritis of the hip causes a great deal of crippling in sufferers who, as a result, become frustrated and very restricted in their activities. For example, they may be unable to do such basic things as wash their feet, cut their toenails, or put on hose or socks without special aids. Walking more than about fifty yards may be excruciatingly painful. Even in bed there is no respite; a chance movement can, by causing pain, wake them at night.

TREATMENT

Operations for the Hip

Ten years ago in affluent countries — as even today in developing countries — the fate of the patient with severe osteoarthritis of both hips was pitiable. Sufferers were in constant pain and very seriously handicapped. Although operations might have relieved pain, they tended to leave the patient with an unpleasant limp.

One of the greatest revolutions in the modern treatment of arthritic and rheumatic diseases has been the development of special hip operations known technically as total hip replacement arthroplasty. These were developed primarily by British surgeons and consist in replacing the hip joints with artificial metal and plastic joints which are glued with special cement into the patients' own living bones.

When the operation is successful the artificial joint functions practically as

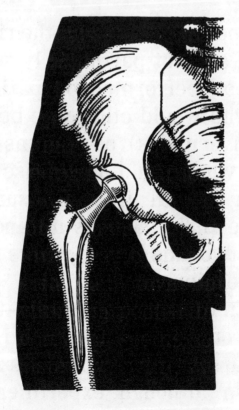

Total hip replacement

well as a natural hip. For those who have been in pain for years a new hip can represent a new life.

How long will they last? Tests show that the artificial hip should last about fifteen or more years of vigorous life before it needs to be replaced, but for many old and frail patients, or those with trouble in other joints, the strain on the joint is likely to be less. In such cases the life of the artificial joint will exceed that of the patient.

With modern anesthetics the risks of the operation are not particularly severe and it has been performed on patients over ninety (who would otherwise be helpless, bedridden cripples) as well as in young children who would otherwise have no hope of a normal life. Most surgeons, in fact, have their patients up and walking between two and three weeks after the date of the operation.

As the modern operation in its present form has only been widely used for about seven years, the long-term risks are not yet known although experimental work has been going on since 1955. The overall failure rate is surprisingly low, less than 5 percent, and this includes patients who are considered bad-risk cases due to other diseases.

Other Methods of Treatment

Aspirin may relieve the pain and stiffness of osteoarthritis in mild cases. The dose is important, however, as twelve or more tablets a day may be needed to have an effect. Then there are other standard pain-relieving drugs, including phenylbutazone and indomethacin, which are particularly useful in the case of hip disease but, as it was pointed out in Chapter 4, they all have their snags — in the form of undesirable side effects.

Warmth or heat administered in the same ways as recommended for other forms of rheumatism also helps to alleviate pain. Many joints with osteoarthritis are cold-sensitive and need to be kept warm. So it is that a bandage around the knee, for example, probably provides relief through the warmth it supplies rather than for any other reason.

The same effect can be achieved by using liniments that contain a warming chemical.

Both rest and exercise may be necessary at different times. If the joint suddenly becomes more painful, it should be rested. If the muscles around the joint become weak because of pain and inactivity, a course of exercises from a physical therapist will strengthen them and prevent the additional pain that comes from joint instability. General exercise is necessary, and one good way of getting this is swimming, an activity that does not place much stress on the joints when they are moving. Most important, however, is that the person find a way of life that will not aggravate the condition. He should not engage in activities that make his joints more painful, such as walking up and down stairs too frequently, jumping down from a truck, or carrying heavy loads. People must learn to pace themselves. Those who are overweight should lose the excess pounds.

Local injections of steroid compounds

are seldom used in osteoarthritis, and if given in the knees, can cause more harm than good to many. The joint at the thumb base, however, can be dramatically relieved by such injections.

Local injections of steroid compounds may be used to relieve the acute inflammation of a joint. Too many of these, however, may cause damage to the joint surfaces.

Trouble in the joints at the base of the toes may mean that special shoes have to be purchased. Remember to have them fitted with rubber heels to absorb the shock of heel impact on the floor during walking. Remember also to use a cane, fitted with a modern nonskid rubber tip. It has been calculated that for a patient with osteoarthritis of one hip, due to a leverage effect, up to two thirds of the weight can be taken off the joint by the use of a cane held in the opposite hand.

The Future

Research is attempting to find methods of improving joint function and preventing fatigue failure. For example, both artificial and natural joint lubricants have been tried, but so far with only limited success.

7

Gout and Pseudo-Gout

Gout is a "snob" form of arthritis, more common among the rich, successful, aggressive, and intelligent. Havelock Ellis, studying all the people listed in Britain's *Dictionary of National Biography,* found that among the famous names included there the frequency of gout was ten times that in the country as a whole. The association of gout with newfound affluence is vividly shown by the story of the Maoris in New Zealand, who, when they left their traditional fish and vegetable diet for a Western diet of beef, bread, sugar, and dairy products, showed an alarming tendency to overweight, coronary disease, and, above all, gout, which has become something of a public health problem among them.

Gout is by no means a rare disease. Of the 20 million people in the United States who have arthritis in one form or another, more than one million are victims of gout.

Gout is also an ancient disease. One of the earliest written references to a specific illness is to gout. Hippocrates, the famous Greek physician of the fifth century B.C., described the type of people likely to suffer from this disease with remarkable insight — even if the implications are somewhat tainted by the moral interpretations of his day.

Eunuchs do not take the gout, nor become bald.

A woman does not take the gout unless her menses be stopped.

A young man does not take the gout until he indulges in coitus.

Today the famous aphorisms of Hippocrates have to be taken with a grain of salt, but it is certainly true that gout is rare in eunuchs and in women; and when women do get gout it is usually after the menopause. But the third aphorism is much more likely to refer to Reiter's syndrome (see Chapter 5), which in its postvenereal form frequently attacks the joints of the feet in young men in a manner resembling gout. Hippocrates' third aphorism is usually (and somewhat innocently) thought to mean that a boy does not get gout until after the age of puberty — which is broadly true, although in modern experience gout is fairly rare in men until the late thirties and forties. Surveys of primitive peoples living today have shown that Reiter's syndrome is common among them. The ancient Greeks were both medically primitive and socially promiscuous, and even if intellectually advanced, they had no real way of telling one sort of acute arthritis (Reiter's) in the toes from another (gout).

The word "gout" came from the Latin word *"gutta"* meaning a drop. The theory — characteristic of the humoral theory of diseases at the time — was that drops of "humors" would flow into a joint and by distending it produce acute inflammation.

INFLAMMATION DUE TO CRYSTALS

Reasonable as these observations and theories seemed to be in the context of their age, we now have a more accurate and scientific knowledge of the conditions they were describing and of the relationship between gout and other diseases. True gout cannot exist without the deposition somewhere in the body of the fine, needle-like crystals of a compound of uric acid. These crystals are the signature of gout, so characteristic that if they are present in some material taken from the body when it is examined under the microscope, then the diagnosis *must* be gout, whatever else the patient is suffering. Most forms of rheumatism have nothing to do with crystals, but the lurid advertisement for bath salt cures for rheumatism, which used to show imaginary rheumatic joints packed with agonizingly sharp crystals, have this element of truth in them — that in some forms of rheumatism, including gout, the joints contain small, sharp crystals. And although for most of the time these crystals are quite innocuous (individual crystals are only about the size of a red blood cell), on other occasions they can give rise to very serious pain. Some people with creaking joints think that the creaking and cracking means they have crystals in their joints. This is not so — the vast majority of noises coming out of a joint are due to other causes.

Crystals and crystalline structures are familiar to us all. Sugar, for example, is a very common crystal and in coffee sugar these crystals are grown to a large size so that it is possible to see that each has a definite shape by which it can be recognized. Common salt is also a crystal but it is ground sufficiently small so that it is almost impossible to spot the characteristic crystal shape of salt, although this can easily be recognized under a low-power microscope. Crystals which are known to cause gout and joint pain in man, however, are very small indeed and can only be seen with certainty under the highest power of the light microscope, while some (hydroxyapatite crystals — see the section on pseudo-gout) are so small that the crystalline structure can only be recognized by X-ray diffraction.

It is only in the last few years that doctors have realized that crystals can be responsible for other types of arthritis as well as for gout, and these other types are listed under pseudo-gout.

In the joint these tiny crystals can be engulfed by certain white blood cells. Also within these cells, there are microscopic bags called lysosomes which contain very powerful substances called enzymes. Enzymes are the factories of the cell, the means whereby it breaks down foreign substances which may penetrate its walls, and the means whereby (in tiny, controlled amounts) it builds up the other substances needed for its life. Unfortunately the cell finds the crystals indigestible. The lysosomes and their enzymes, instead of dissolving the crystals, are burst by them, with the result that the enzymes are liberated within the cell (which may die) and then into the joint, where they produce severe inflammation. The most well-known form of crystal-induced inflammation in the joint is gout. The particular inducing agent is crystals of uric acid, a relatively insoluble chemical that is deposited from the blood. The same type of acute inflammation can also be induced by other crystals.

Pseudo-gout, as its name suggests, resembles gout very closely, but is due to crystals of a different chemical derived from lime — calcium pyrophosphate.

Identification of the Crystals

How, therefore, do we discover and identify these crystals? This is a highly technical procedure but it can be readily undertaken in the laboratory by a trained technician. The crystals of gout and pseudo-gout are different and can be distinguished by specific optical properties.

GOUT — A RICH MAN'S DISEASE?

It is commonly thought that gout is a disease of the well-to-do. The word itself elicits the image of the exquisitely dressed Regency gentleman quietly sipping his port, resting an enormous bandaged foot on a foot stool. Special gout footstools on which to rest the painful foot were once made, adjustable to the correct height. They are now collectors' items.

Gout can affect any member of the population but, as Hippocrates said, gout is more common in men than women, and usually starts in young middle-aged males, whereas in women it only commences after about fifty years of age. Very, very rarely, true gout occurs in children. Certain forms of pseudo-gout (caused by crystals other than uric acid) are more frequent in teen-agers.

Types of Gout

True uric acid gout passes through two phases. Initially there is an acute stage, in which the subject suffers from recurrent attacks of severe and often painful arthritis, very often in the big toe joint. After each attack the toe seems to return completely to normal — until the next bout. But after a number of attacks, the chronic stage is reached. The joint gets progressively more damaged; it does not completely return to normal between attacks but fluctuates between relatively painless deformity and relatively painful inflammation.

Acute gout Of all the pains known to man, acute gout can be among the worst. In a bad attack, the joint becomes intensely swollen, inflamed, and excruciatingly painful; it is so tender that the sufferer cannot bear even the slightest pressure to be placed upon it. The old joke says, "If one of your friends took a large pair of pliers and squeezed the big toe joint hard — that's arthritis. But if one of your *enemies* did it, then that's gout."

Without treatment the attack usually lasts for a few days and then slowly recedes.

Why is it that gout usually starts in the joint of the big toe? There is no fully proved explanation, but it seems likely that there are two main reasons. The first is that the big toe joint often shows osteoarthritis (damage due to wear and tear) before all other joints, even in young people, presumably because of the effect of shoes. The second is that the big toe joint, being the joint farthest from the heart, is also the coldest joint in the body. These two factors, local damage — which is usually associated with local acidity of joint fluid — plus the lower temperature, both favor the crystallization of uric acid from its solution in the blood.

Chronic gout Repeated attacks of acute gout eventually produce permanent damage because uric acid crystals sooner or later destroy the joint surfaces. The joint becomes filled with large masses of crystals that look like chalk. It appears to be very swollen, and movements are limited and painful. It is also possible for an acute attack to occur where chronic joint damage already exists.

Gout mainly tends to damage the big toe joint, but destruction of the joints can also occur in the fingers, elbows, and elsewhere.

Uric acid may be deposited in other tissues. It is often found in skin on the backs of the elbows, on the margins of the ears, and in the hands. Collections of uric acid crystals appear just beneath the surface and can sometimes burst through the skin producing ulcers which discharge white chalky material.

Gout and the Kidneys

The kidney is another part of the body that can be damaged by uric acid. In fact, for practical purposes, it is the only internal organ of the body which is commonly damaged by urate crystals. Collections of crystals of uric acid accumulate in the kidney and in time can gradually destroy it.

Kidney damage is probably more serious in the long run than joint damage. Painful joints can make life miserable from time to time, but damaged kidneys threaten life itself, either directly because they fail to get rid of waste products, or indirectly because they lead to high blood pressure which in turn may lead to heart disease and stroke. Even when kidney damage is not too severe, it still has unfortunate results since uric acid itself is one of the waste products of the body and is normally eliminated by the kidneys into the urine (hence its name). If the kidney, damaged by gout, becomes even less efficient at getting rid of uric acid, then this makes the condition worse.

Uric Acid

The problems of gout center around the formation and removal of uric acid. If you make too much of it, or if you fail to get rid of it, then the waste accumulates in the body and the result, sooner or later, is gout.

It is by no means the case that all the uric acid in the body comes from the diet. Some is produced by the building up and breaking down that goes on within all the cells in the body — muscle cells, liver cells, blood cells; all are being continuously manufactured to replace worn-out cells. Biologists speak of this as cell turnover, much as a shopkeeper, stocking up his shelves and emptying them again, would talk about his turnover. Part of the uric acid in the body results from this normal cell turnover. But in certain blood conditions, such as polycythemia (too many red cells) and in skin conditions, such as psoriasis, the amount of cell turnover is greatly increased; thus people with these diseases are particularly susceptible to gout.

Part of the uric acid in the body comes from the cells in the food we eat, and foods that contain high concentrations of cells are traditionally liable to bring on gout. The principal foods are liver, kidneys, sweetbreads, brains, meat extracts, fish roes, anchovies, and sardines. However, this list is not exclusive.

The third way in which uric acid is manufactured in the body is by direct chemical synthesis, without being built up into the proteins of the cells. A man who eats no meat, fish, or organs but who gets all his protein in the form of cheese, will still produce more uric acid than a man existing on a purely vegetarian diet. Furthermore, it is not just the type of food that matters, but also the amount consumed.

So much for the ways in which uric acid is made in the body. If any one of these methods of manufacture is working overtime, gout may result. But gout may also be developed if the methods of manufacture are all working at normal speed, but the methods of getting rid of uric acid begin to fail. Some of the body's uric acid is disposed of in the skin and some by passing into the digestive juices in the bowel where it meets bacteria that are capable of breaking it down. Up to one third of the uric acid produced is eliminated in these ways.

But by far the largest amount of uric acid passes by a complicated route through the kidneys and is excreted in the urine. People with large quantities of uric acid in the body who lose excessive amounts through the kidneys may develop kidney stones and renal colic.

We have already seen how kidney damage can cause the kidneys to be less efficient at getting rid of uric acid, but it is not the only factor. People who drink alcohol burn it, just as sugar is burned in the body to provide energy. But alcohol is not just burned in the same way that it would burn in an alcohol lamp. In the body it passes through the stage of transformation to lactic acid. People who drink quantities of alcohol have a lot of lactic acid in their blood, and lactic acid can affect the kidneys and stop them from getting rid of uric acid. The greater the alcohol intake, the less uric acid is eliminated. It is easy to see that people who eat well (producing more uric acid) and who drink well (disposing of less uric acid) are those who are candidates for gout.

Aspirin (acetylsalicylic acid) is one of a number of slightly acid drugs which also have the power to influence the rate of elimination of uric acid, and this is why people with gout should not take aspirin for headaches. There are other important drugs, such as some diuretics used for reducing excessive fluids in the body, that may interfere with the elimination of uric acid via the kidneys and therefore cause gout.

The other key to the understanding of the role of uric acid in gout lies in its solubility. Uric acid circulates in the blood in the form of its poorly soluble salt, sodium biurate. If warm blood is shaken up with uric acid in a test tube, for example, the maximum amount that will dissolve is only about 6 mg. in 100 cc. But blood is traditionally thicker than water, and the thickness is due to plasma proteins which are able to keep uric acid in solution at levels far above the natural solubility. Because of this, all persons with gout, unless they are on treatment, have more (and sometimes two to three times as much) uric acid in the blood than is desirable because of simple solubility. In chemical terms their blood is a supersaturated solution of uric acid, and as any chemist will tell you, a supersaturated solution is one that can very easily be made to deposit crystals.

So it is with uric acid crystals. In

persons with gout there is a strong tendency to form crystals, and for local reasons the tendency is strongest in the joints and kidneys. As long as a supersaturated solution occurs, crystallization will continue.

In the past, before there were any effective treatments, some unfortunate sufferers would accumulate as much as half a pound of solid uric acid on and about their bodies. Enormous white chalky lumps could be seen. Today, with effective treatments, most medical students in training will never see gout as bad as that — they will only read about it.

The solubility of uric acid in blood is also a clue to the cure of gout. If the amount of uric acid dissolved in the blood can be kept down below about 6 mg. in 100 cc., then crystals of uric acid will steadily dissolve back again into the blood. And as we will see later in this chapter, this can be made to happen.

TREATMENT

Eating . . .

If gout is associated with rich living, then treatment must surely imply that a rather more spartan life-style is needed. However, mainly because of the miracles of modern medicine, this is not so. There are certain protein foods — listed on page 111 — that have a high concentration of cells and therefore have a high potential for forming uric acid in the body. It would seem wise to avoid eating them where possible. But in fact, the drug treatment of gout is now so effective that it is hardly necessary to impose severe dietary restrictions on patients, other than the common-sense one that if a person is obviously overeating and overdrinking, he should bring this down to sensible levels. If gout can be controlled without having to be a martyr to a special diet, so much the better.

. . . And Drinking

It is valuable to drink plenty of fluid such as water, tea, or coffee. Five or six pints a day will increase the flow of urine considerably and will help prevent kidney damage or the appearance of stones.

However, the above advice should not provide an excuse for the gouty subject to disappear to his neighborhood bar every night for the recommended five or six pints of fluid — alcohol is certainly not a part of the cure! Gout and alcohol are traditionally associated with each other and there is some justification for this. Bartenders, hoteliers, and brewery workers, for whom alcohol is an occupational hazard; stockbrokers, bankers, and salesmen, who are exposed to the necessity of frequent business lunches; and others who live well, such as businessmen and, let it be admitted, doctors, all have occupations whose members have more gout than do other more abstemious groups.

But alcohol is not related to gout only because of lactic acid's effect on the kidneys. In the days before there was proper control of pollution, lead workers were especially liable to gout because lead damaged the kidneys. Even today, people who distill illicit moonshine whiskey may get very severe gout, not because of the alcohol, but because of the lead in it due to contamination from the old lead piping, etc., from which they make their do-it-yourself stills.

There is one other way in which alcoholic drinks can affect gout. Some people, already gouty, find themselves sensitive to certain types of wine. For them champagne, perhaps, or port, can regularly bring on an attack, whereas a whiskey and water, containing the same amount of alcohol, would have no such effect. Port in particular has a specially bad reputation for producing acute attacks, but other wines may be equally responsible.

But the real issue about alcohol is not the kind of drink consumed — it is the amount. As with all other things in life, moderation in drinking alcohol is the correct advice.

Treating the Acute Attack

Gout is one of those diseases that seem to have suffered from an old precept that the more a treatment hurts, the more good it is doing. In the past, acute gout was so painful that extreme types of treatment were used in order to relieve the symptoms. Unfortunately these methods were not based upon an accurate knowledge of the disease; terrifying cures such as cutting the skin over the joint with a knife, applying burning compresses, or blistering the skin over the joint were common. Indeed the treatment was often worse than the disease. But because an acute attack of gout usually only lasts two or three days the subsequent relief was seen as evidence of the value of the treatment.

Today treatment is rather more civilized as well as more effective. The most common drugs used are colchicine, indomethacin, and phenylbutazone. When taken in correct amounts they will relieve the severe pain in only a few hours.

Colchicine is a drug with an interesting history. The Byzantine physicians in Constantinople discovered that a particular substance extracted from the autumn crocus provided an effective form of treatment. It was subsequently used in Europe up to about the thirteenth century when, somehow, colchicine became lost to medicine. It was not rediscovered until the late eighteenth century, and it was gout-sufferer Benjamin Franklin who is credited with the introduction of the drug in America. The autumn crocus has been responsible for providing relief to many gout sufferers, but it is becoming obsolete since modern drugs are more effective and on the whole their adverse effects are less troublesome.

Gout and aspirin, however, do not mix. Aspirin in all its forms and in the proprietary mixtures that may be purchased at the drugstore are to be avoided in treating gout. This is because aspirin affects the complicated pathways by which uric acid is lost from the body through the kidneys. Instead of helping the situation it may do the exact opposite, by actually reducing the loss of uric acid from the body.

Advising a person suffering from a severe attack of gout to rest is like telling a man without legs not to walk. The joint is so painful that the subject is not capable of anything but resting. People with milder attacks, however, need this advice because walking around will usually make them worse. When the big toe joint is affected, resting in bed can only be effective if the foot is protected from the weight of the bedclothes. A specially designed device will lift the clothes off the foot, but if this is not available, a large cardboard box with two sides cut out of it will suffice.

Treating Chronic Gout

The drugs used for acute gout (colchicine, indomethacin, and phenylbutazone) do nothing to reduce the amount of uric acid in the body. Although they relieve gout's pain, they will not prevent further attacks in the future, nor will they alter any uric acid deposits in the skin, joints, or kidneys.

However, in recent years, a fuller understanding of the complicated pathway by which uric acid is formed and removed has led to the development of effective drugs designed to reduce the amount of uric acid in the body. These drugs are of two types:

1. Drugs that reduce the formation of uric acid, such as allopurinol

2. Drugs that increase the loss of uric acid through the kidney, such as probenecid

Once it is necessary to start taking these drugs, it is almost always essential to continue the treatment throughout life. To put it simply, if bluntly, treatment for gout is treatment for life. Fresh attacks of gout will be prevented and the joint swellings, the damage to joints seen on X-ray, and the visible deposits of uric acid in the skin will heal.

Unfortunately, during the first few weeks of treatment, these drugs may actually stir up the gout. The reason for this is not at all clear, but it seems that they exert such a profound influence in moving uric acid from the deposits, where it is relatively harmless, that free uric acid becomes available and gets into new, sensitive areas. There is a danger here which a patient does not readily understand. If he takes a drug for gout and it seems to make his gout worse, why should he persist? Obviously he won't think much of the new treatment unless the problem is explained to him and he is warned in advance. However, this is a problem that need not dismay those who want a long-term cure for gout; these initial painful attacks can be prevented by taking small doses of the acute attack drugs during the first couple of months of treatment with the chronic gout drugs.

Today, gout should be completely controlled and the motto should be "There can be no excuse for gout."

Research into Gout

Gout is perhaps the best example in rheumatology of how research can lead to effective control of a disease. Improved understanding of the complex way in which uric acid is formed and lost from the body has led to the development of specific drugs and to the present satisfactory situation. Nevertheless, knowledge is never complete and there is still a lot more work in progress aimed at pinpointing the various biochemical problems that initiate gout, and at defining specific abnormalities to enable us to have an even better understanding of the disease.

PSEUDO-GOUT: CHONDROCALCINOSIS

Uric acid is not the only crystalline substance that can produce acute joint inflammation. For many years doctors have recognized that there is a special form of arthritis due to chalk-like substances other than uric acid being deposited in the joints. This material was later discovered to be a crystalline form of a substance derived from lime — calcium pyrophosphate. The similarities of the inflammation induced by this chemical to that induced by uric acid are reflected in one of its names — pseudo-gout. It is also called calcium gout and another name, which is perhaps rather more difficult to remember, is chondrocalcinosis. The reason for this second name — "chondro" refers to the cartilage and "calcinosis" means calcium.

Chondrocalcinosis can affect adults at almost any age, the only distinctive feature being that it sometimes runs in families.

Characteristically, it is the knee joint that is affected by this condition but it can also occur elsewhere, such as the wrist, elbow, hip, shoulder, or spine. The trouble usually becomes apparent because of repeated attacks of severe arthritis, which can be as painful as in acute gout. Sometimes, however, the condition produces chronic wear and tear — or osteoarthritis — and then the symptoms take the form of aches and pains and a feeling of grating in the joint.

It is the X-ray that provides the clue to the diagnosis. This shows the abnormal chalky material and leads the doctor to examine some of the joint fluid under the polarizing microscope. The particular crystals of calcium pyrophosphate will then be discovered.

Although no one really knows why, chondrocalcinosis sometimes coincides with other diseases. Unfortunately, treatment of these diseases does not relieve the arthritis.

Treatment

Aspirin, indomethacin, phenylbutazone, and other similar drugs are usually effective, severe pain subsiding within one or two days. It may be helpful to take small amounts of these drugs continuously to prevent any relapse.

Research

Normally calcium pyrophosphate is destroyed by a particular enzyme. Recent research has shown that this enzyme is missing in persons with this condition so that calcium pyrophosphate accumulates and is deposited in the joint.

PERIARTICULAR CALCIFICATION

Periarticular calcification is another form of crystal gout in which a different chemical — calcium hydroxyapatite — is involved. In contrast with pseudo-gout, this substance is deposited in the soft tissues around the joint, but not actually in the joint lining. Inflammation is produced in precisely the same way. Whereas chondrocalcinosis affects old people, with sufferers usually in their sixties and seventies or more, periarticular calcification is more often seen in young adults, and occasionally even in children.

8

Soft Tissue Rheumatism

In a book of this nature, one would assume that the most relevant or, rather, the more interesting information would perhaps be about those numerous minor but nevertheless painful conditions that most of us suffer from at various times in our lives. Few people visit the doctor to complain of having a stiff neck, a stitch or cramp, nor do they feel it necessary to see him because of aches and pains which they know by experience will disappear when, for example, they are less tense or perhaps when the cold winter is over. So, while the other conditions so far described in this book will have been explained — if only briefly — to the patients by their doctors, most of us remain ignorant about these more general, less serious conditions.

This chapter will therefore deal, in some detail, with many of these soft tissue types of rheumatism.

The distinction between soft tissue and hard tissue is this: rheumatism in hard tissues refers to the various well-known, well-defined, and sometimes serious cases of arthritis that arise in the joints and bones of the limbs and spine (such as are described in the previous chapters). Soft tissue rheumatism refers to a very large group of miscellaneous and ill-defined painful conditions that seem to arise in the fleshy parts.

Therefore, although none of the conditions about to be described in this chapter necessarily relate to each other (that is, if you have one kind of soft tissue rheumatism, it does not necessarily mean that you are liable to get the others), they do have one common feature which is that they all seem to arise in the soft tissues of the body.

These particular types of aches and pains are indisputably common. For instance, in Britain in 1968, when the figures were last available, soft tissue rheumatism of one sort or another caused a loss of 10 million work days to industry and each worker affected lost an average of twenty-two days per year. Ironic as it may sound, if one considers this staggering total in relation to the number of days lost each year due to industrial disputes, rheumatic illnesses of this type represent as large a problem to the economy as do strikes. And, enormous as the total is, it certainly does not justly represent the frequency of these conditions, since many of the sufferers continue to work and others are housewives and retired people who remain uncounted. The problem is so common that everyone will have soft tissue rheumatism in one form or another at some time in his life. Some forms, such as cramp and stitch, are universal, mild, and hardly disabling. Other kinds are serious and quite crippling.

There are two types of soft tissue rheumatism:

1. Generalized, that is, affecting many parts of the body

2. Localized, which means arising in one or two areas only

GENERALIZED SOFT TISSUE RHEUMATISM

These conditions affect people who "ache all over" or who after resting seem to stiffen up so much that they feel pain when attempting to move about again.

Doctors who deal with rheumatic conditions have to be on their guard with this type of complaint, since as we know by experience, generalized aching is sometimes the way in which non-rheumatic diseases begin. Influenza, as an obvious example, often begins as aching in the neck, shoulders, and back. However, blood tests and X-rays (or just a few days of observation) usually will enable the doctor to give a clear diagnosis.

Fibrositis

Fibrositis, as you may remember, has already been referred to briefly in Chapter 1 as nonspecific back pain, and in Chapter 3 as a cervical fibrositis, where a general ignorance as to its exact cause was confessed.

The word itself — fibrositis — is no longer a medical term despite its official-sounding name. It refers to aching and tenderness in the muscles, particularly those at the back of the neck and head, and in the soft parts at the top of the shoulder. It is also sometimes used with reference to a similar type of aching where the muscles of the low back join the pelvis.

Although fibrositis is extremely common, particularly in the neck, people vary tremendously in terms of how frequently they suffer from it and the type of conditions that initiate it. Certain factors tend to aggravate the pain for particular people: some people only suffer from it when they are ill, tense, tired, or worried, others when they are chilled or have been in a draft. Some people only get it while they are developing a cold, and some unfortunate people suffer all the time. One of the commonest causes is sleeping soundly with the head and neck in an awkward position because of the height of the pillows. Children seldom suffer from this because of the suppleness of their necks, but it is particularly important for old people to have a pillow that is exactly right to allow for the stiffness of their necks.

Fibrositis is not a disabling condition and is in fact rarely more than a recurrent nuisance. If it does become more prolonged and incapacitating, then more intensive treatment is required. Temporary relief of fibrositis is gained either by rubbing the painful area or by applying heat or liniments that contain something that generates a feeling of warmth. However, Chapter 3 has already dealt extensively with the treatment of the painful neck.

One warning worth mentioning, though, is about frequent massage. What happens is that massage provides temporary relief, but much of the deep massage, which is sometimes given very forcibly, bruises the muscles. Not surprisingly therefore, the trouble now heightened, the patient returns the following day requiring more massage — and so the story goes on.

Polymyalgia Rheumatica

This is a disease of the elderly, and sometimes of the not so elderly.

Polymyalgia rheumatica is one of the commonest causes of generalized soft tissue rheumatism after the age of sixty-five. As a cause of rheumatism, it is at least as common as gout and affects about one in every hundred people of that age group.

The onset of this disease is often quite sudden, affecting older people who up till then have been remarkably fit and vigorous for their age. The sufferer feels generally ill and complains of pain in the neck, back, shoulders, and thighs, though thankfully not all at the same time. The striking characteristic of this condition is the way in which the afflicted person stiffens up after resting. This is particularly bad in the mornings; in fact it is sometimes so severe that he is practically paralyzed for an hour or more until the stiffening eases up.

A middle-aged person who gets polymyalgia rheumatica usually feels that he has become prematurely old; an old person often thinks his life is at an end. However, treatment in most cases is ridiculously simple. A few tablets of prednisone produce an apparently miraculous cure after only a few days or even sometimes after a few hours. This particular drug was discussed in Chapter 4, where it was pointed out that prednisone — a derivative of cortisone — is not without dangers. This source of a new lease on life must only be taken under medical supervision and according to the results of regular blood tests.

The cause of polymyalgia rheumatica is unknown. It is not a disease of the muscles even though that is where the pain is felt. Sometimes it is associated with a disease in the arteries called temporal arteritis; this is a potentially serious condition which, by blocking vital arteries in the eye or head, can lead to blindness or a stroke. Again prednisone acts as a "magical" drug in preventing this.

A similar but extremely rare condition in younger people is caused by direct inflammation of the muscles and is called polymyositis. The similarity is only in the symptoms — weakness, stiffness, and a general tenderness of the muscles.

Other Causes of Generalized Soft Tissue Rheumatism

There are many other types and causes of soft tissue rheumatism. The following list shows some of the strange assortment of factors that can cause this generalized aching and pain:

1. The commonest cause perhaps is the aching and tenderness in the back and the limbs that some people get when they put on weight rapidly.

2. Older people who become "hooked" on sleeping tablets sometimes develop

generalized aching.

3. Some younger women get similar aching when they take the contraceptive pill.

4. Some people develop aching after unaccustomed exercise.

LOCALIZED SOFT TISSUE RHEUMATISM

Localized soft tissue rheumatism is a convenient term for grouping all the different pains, strains, and aches that arise and are felt in a specific area due to a particular type of damage or strain on a part of the soft tissue.

The types of soft tissue rheumatism that will now be explained can be divided into groups according to the particular tissue affected:

1. Strained or sprained ligaments
2. Tensed muscles
3. Damage to the shoulder joint
4. Inflammation or damage to the bursa (bursitis)
5. Swelling of the carpal tunnel in the wrist.

6. Swelling of the tendons (tendinitis)

7. Damage to the enthesis (tennis elbow, etc.)

Strains and Sprains

Strain occurs when a ligament is stretched. The ligaments or check straps limit movement in a joint. Therefore, if a joint is forced in a direction that it cannot bend, the particular ligaments stopping this impossible movement become stretched.

An example will perhaps clarify this process: a person who goes to sleep in a railway carriage with his feet up on the opposite seat will awaken to find that his knees feel stiff and painful. This is because the whole weight of his leg has been hanging on the ligaments at the back of the knee, and it is only they, not his muscles, that have prevented the joint from bending back to front. These ligaments have been strained. Similarly, the gardener who is weeding a garden is "hanging on his back" all day, and so may strain ligaments in his back. A patient

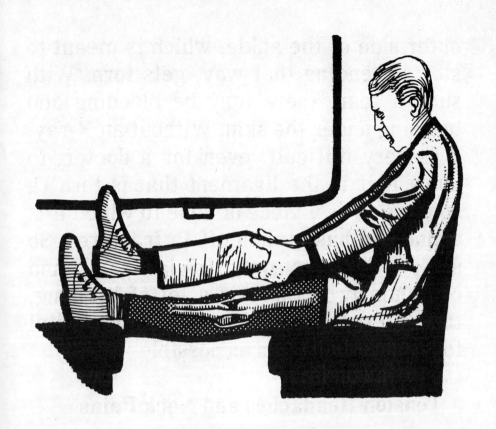

who has suffered a stroke so that one arm is paralyzed will often experience severe pain in the shoulder joint because the whole weight of the paralyzed arm is hanging on the joint without any protection by the muscles.

A sprain, on the other hand, is a torn ligament. The most familiar example is the sprained ankle and the most common way of doing it is to run downstairs, miss one's footing, and land so as forcibly to twist the foot inward. The ligament at the outer side of the ankle, which is meant to stop it bending that way, gets torn. With such a tear, there may be bleeding and bruising under the skin. Without an X-ray, it is very difficult, even for a doctor, to know if it is the ligament that is torn (a sprain), or if a piece of bone to which it is connected has broken off (a fracture). So unless there is only trivial pain, and particularly if there is a lot of bruising, the sufferer should always go to a hospital for an X-ray as soon as possible.

Tension Headaches and Neck Pains

Most of the muscles in the body relax completely when they are not being used. But some muscles, known as the antigravity muscles, must work all the time in order to keep the body upright. For example, the jaw muscles must never relax, for if they did, the mouth would fall open (as it does when a person falls asleep while sitting in a chair). Similarly, the muscles at the back of the neck must always be tensed, otherwise the head would fall forward when a person was

236

sitting or standing.

Tension headaches are often part of the problem of fibrositis. When people are worried they often tighten their muscles more than is necessary to hold the head upright. In other words, they are literally tense and this in turn generates a strain on the places where the muscles are attached to the back of the head. The muscle attachments become tender and painful, and when the pain is severe it will spread from the back of the head and neck, upward and forward over the head until it seems to be behind the eyes.

These tension headaches are very

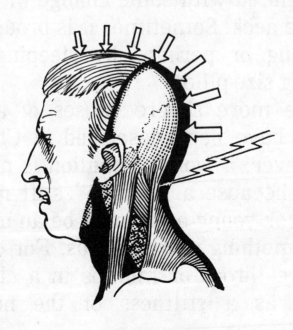

common and are often — wrongly — called migraine by patients. The answer to them is usually quite simple: take a painkiller such as aspirin — a small dose of this will suffice — and get into a warm bed. A few minutes' sleep will allow the antigravity muscles at the back of the neck to relax and, miraculously, the headache will normally disappear.

A stiff neck is another common form of soft tissue rheumatism which is usually generated by tensed muscles. The muscles involved are again at the back of the neck, but are lower down than those that cause tension headaches. It is often associated with some change in the discs of the neck. Sometimes it is brought on by chilling or perhaps by sleeping on the wrong size pillow.

The more severe causes of a painful neck have been described in Chapter 3. However, a word of caution is necessary here because a "simple" stiff neck in a child or young adult may be an indication of something more serious. For example, a sore throat or mumps in a child may start as a stiffness of the neck, the stiffening in this case being due to swelling and pain in the glands of the neck. There will usually be fever as well. More sinister causes of a stiff neck in childhood are meningitis and polio, where the stiffness is due to inflammation of the spinal cord rather than the neck muscles.

In young adults, there is a particular form of stiffness called wry neck or torticollis; in this condition there is such muscle spasm that the neck is not only stiff but the head is pulled to one side. Treatment can take a long time, and as the cause is not known, the condition is not easily curable and can be quite disabling. The unfortunate sufferer often notices that the neck spasm and twisting are worse when any work is attempted.

The Painful Shoulder*

Shoulder pains are common; ironically, however, most of these pains come from the neck. There is a simple distinction

---

* Not included in this category are the stiff painful shoulders caused by polymyalgia rheumatica, from

239

between true shoulder pain and pain felt in the shoulder but actually arising from the neck; if it is difficult or painful to *move* the shoulder joint, then the trouble is arising from the shoulder — an obvious fact that is rarely recognized.

Painful shoulders are sometimes due to trouble in the acromioclavicular joint — a little joint that connects the collarbone to the shoulder blade. Damage to this joint is a common sports injury but can often be relieved rapidly by injection.

Another type of shoulder pain is due to a peculiar condition called capsulitis of the shoulder. The popular name for this is frozen shoulder. It affects people in the forty-to-sixty age range and often results in very uncomfortable and disturbed sleep. It is impossible, not just painful, for the sufferer to raise his arm high. The frustrations are obvious — women cannot even hang clothes on the line, and men find that they cannot reach things from a

which elderly people suffer. A blood test will indicate whether polymyalgia rheumatica is the cause, or whether it is purely a shoulder joint problem.

high shelf. Frozen shoulder may persist for many months, and often requires physical therapy or manipulation under an anesthetic before it gets better.

But by far the commonest painful condition of the shoulder is bursitis — a form of soft tissue rheumatism. This will be dealt with in the next category along with the other conditions that develop as a result of some types of trouble with a bursa.

Bursitis

The bursa is the medical name for the space between a soft part of the body, usually a tendon or a muscle, and the place where it rubs over a bone or joint. Its purpose is to lubricate this gliding surface (and so improve the efficiency of the body as a machine). But, as with all machines, something can go wrong. A bursa can become rough or inflamed or even fill with fluid. It has a lining that is similar to that of a joint, so it can also be affected by joint diseases such as rheumatoid arthritis or gout.

Bursitis of the shoulder Bursitis of the shoulder is due to an inflammation of the bursa that cushions the motions of the joint. The onset of this condition tends to occur after the age of forty in most patients. The characteristic feature is that, although it is possible to raise the hand high above the head, as the arm is dropped downward and sideways, pain develops over the middle range of movement and then disappears when the arm is allowed to fall to the side. Happily, however, it can often be relieved rapidly by medicines or injection treatments.

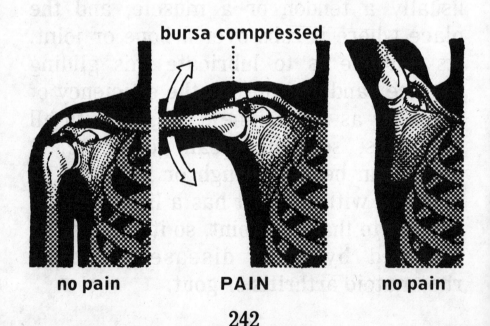

bursa compressed

no pain　　　**PAIN**　　　**no pain**

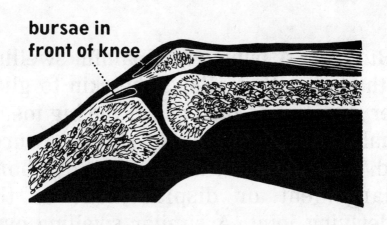

bursae in front of knee

Housemaid's knee, beat elbow These may sound a strange collection of medical names but the meaning of each is fairly obvious, if not altogether self-explanatory.

In housemaid's knee, the bursa affected is the one that allows the skin to glide over the kneecap while a person is kneeling. Continuous pressure often causes it to become inflamed; this naturally affected housemaids who scrubbed floors by kneeling on the floor and scrubbing with a brush. Similarly it would affect nuns, or miners before the days of automatic coal-cutting machinery, when it was a common industrial injury known as beat knee. Beat elbow is a similar form of bursitis affecting the point of the elbow.

Bunion A bunion is a painful swelling in the bursa that allows the skin to glide over the joint at the base of the big toe. It usually swells because of shoe pressures and is often made worse by bony enlargement or displacement of the underlying joint. A similar swelling over the base of the little toe is known as a bunionette.*

Snapping shoulder and snapping hip These are conditions which, amazingly, often start as a type of party trick, but then become a habit. In snapping shoulder the person finds that he can make a loud snapping noise by hunching his shoulder blade in a certain way. The noise arises from underneath the shoulder blade where it rubs over the muscles and ribs. However, there is a bursa in this spot that eventually becomes inflamed and painful. Snapping the shoulder seems to relieve the pain

* See Chapter 10 for information about rheumatism of the foot.

244

temporarily, but only perpetuates the condition.

In snapping hip the trouble is similar, but the snapping there is caused by a flat tendon that slips over the prominence of the hip during walking.

Carpal tunnel syndrome When you clench your hand you can see a number of tendons passing from the muscles in the arms to the fingers; the tunnel through which they pass between the bones in front of the wrist is called the carpal tunnel. The lining of this is similar to a bursa, and, like the bursa, it may become inflamed and swollen. The problem of this swelling is increased by the fact that an important nerve — the median nerve — passes through this same tunnel to the hand and there is no room to spare. The swelling therefore immediately places pressure on this nerve, and if the pressure is great, the nerve cannot conduct messages so that the index, middle, and half of the ring finger will become numb. Pressure is seldom bad enough to block this nerve altogether, but it does

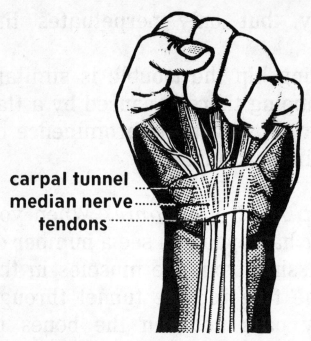

carpal tunnel
median nerve
tendons

The carpal tunnel

cause irritation and severe pain. Characteristically, the pain, which has a special burning quality, spreads throughout the hand and arm when the pressure is severe. It is usually much worse at night, and sufferers often describe how they hang their hands outside the bedclothes in an attempt to get some relief by cooling them.

Carpal tunnel syndrome is quite frequent in early rheumatoid arthritis, but most cases have nothing to do with any generalized form of arthritis. Attacks usually develop because of gradual thickening of the soft tissue in the front of the tunnel at the wrist as the subject gets older. Middle-aged women are most frequently affected, and the problem is particularly common at menopause. However, it also occurs in men from time to time and is a well-known complication in younger women when they are pregnant. Relief can usually be obtained by a wrist splint or by injecting a little hydrocortisone into the tunnel, but some patients will require a minor operation to take the pressure off the sensitive nerve.

Tendonitis

The tendon is the string or leader that connects a muscle to a bone. Painful inflammation in the tendon is known as tendinitis, and a common area for this is on the thumb side of the wrist where one of the thumb tendons winds around the forearm bone. Another common place is at the back of the heel where the powerful calf muscles are attached. Inside the hand the swelling of a tendon, or a lump forming on the tendon, may give rise to trigger finger. The lump will not slide past a constriction in its tunnel. This condition — as suggested by its name — becomes evident to the patient when he notices that the finger can be bent but then won't straighten unless actively pushed back with the other hand, when it then straightens with a snap. Skilled hand surgeons can relieve a trigger finger with a minor operation.

Enthesitis

The enthesis is the place where the muscle or tendon is joined onto a bone; it is also the area in which the pain nerve fibers are particularly numerous.

The generalized stiffness and pain that affect people who are out of training and have been doing some hard exercise are probably due to minor damage to the entheses. But there are two or three specific forms of enthesitis that are very common and persistent causes of soft tissue rheumatism.

Tennis elbow arises where the powerful

forearm muscles join the bone at the outer side of the elbow. Golfer's elbow is similar but affects the inner side of the elbow.

Policeman's heel is a similar condition, but exists beneath the heel. The pelvis is also sometimes affected where some of the powerful leg muscles are joined to the bone.

Inflammation of many entheses occurs in ankylosing spondylitis (Chapter 2) in different sites in the body.

TREATMENT

Almost all local causes of soft tissue rheumatism are treated first with drugs such as aspirin, indomethacin or phenylbutazone and then, if the oral medication fails, by local injections of hydrocortisone, with or without a local anesthetic. This is often very effective, and sometimes only one injection can produce a cure. For difficult or recurrent problems, long-acting derivatives of hydrocortisone are available. Occasionally minor operations are necessary.

FACTORS INCREASING THE DISCOMFORT OF RHEUMATISM

There are certain conditions and factors that seem to increase the occurrence and frequency of soft tissue rheumatism. Cold sensitivity, poor blood supply, and over-supple joints can make people particularly liable to suffer from certain rheumatic conditions.

Cold-Sensitive Rheumatism

Many rheumatic conditions are cold-sensitive, that is, the pain seems to increase in cold, damp weather and decrease in warm, dry weather. This has given rise to the popular belief that rheumatism is more frequent in moist climates (such as in Britain) and almost nonexistent in the Sahara Desert. This is, in fact, a myth; rheumatism is not less common in hot countries, but it does hurt less. Any well-defined type of rheumatism or arthritis — such as rheumatoid arthritis — is as common in the dry parts of the United States as in wet Britain. The reason that some Africans or other members of the less affluent nations suffer less from arthritis than inhabitants of the affluent countries is the shorter life expectancy of the former — they just don't live long enough to get serious rheumatic conditions. However, the myth is understandable, for although immigration into a warmer country will not change the fundamental cause of arthritis, it *will* make the condition seem less painful, which, after all, is what the sufferer is concerned about.

But emigration to another part of the world with a warmer, drier climate has its disadvantages, and for many the costs of making the move may outweigh any benefits. There are simpler methods of dealing with sensitivity to cold — which is often particularly intense for sufferers from low back pain — such as placing a hot water bottle on the back. Any cold draft or chilling may increase the pain, and for some sufferers it may be impossible to get to sleep without a hot water bottle on the back, even in

251

the summer.

Similar cold-sensitive pain occurs around the knee, particularly in women, where one sometimes finds pads of discolored fat that are tender and cold to the touch. They may be one or two degrees cooler in temperature than the surrounding area when tested with a special thermometer.

Cold-sensitive rheumatism is best treated with a close-fitting warm garment, as countless generations of hardworking peasants who do back-breaking work have found out. In Poland they wear rabbit skins on the back; in southern France, Spain, and Italy, wide woolen cummerbunds are part of the national peasant dress. In England, Doll's flannel is the traditional thing for a working man's backache, and modern equivalents include insulating thermal underwear.

Loose Joints: An Asset or Liability?

Just as people vary in height, weight, hair, complexion, and so on, so do they also vary in the suppleness and stiffness of their joints. There is just as much variation of agility in people as between racehorses and carthorses, greyhounds and bulldogs. Indians and Arabs tend to have suppler joints than people of Western European stock, but there is a good deal of individual variation within each race. Children are more supple than adults, and adults are more supple than old people. But with constant training and practice, a dancer or athlete can keep the joints more supple than his or her contemporaries, even to the age of sixty or more.

However, some kinds of suppleness seem to be harmful and lead to injuries to joints and the soft tissues. Indeed in some, suppleness is so severe that patients with it are defined as having definite diseases, running in the family. An example is Marfan's syndrome; the affected person usually has very long fingers and toes and legs — quite disproportionately long in comparison to the height of the trunk. The muscles in this condition are relatively weak and the ligaments are so slack that the spine and joints can easily become deformed, dislocated, or damaged.

But lesser degrees of hyperlaxity exist and may be partly an asset as well as partly a liability. For example, in a study of American football players it was discovered that an above-average number of players had an unusual laxity of the joints. In other words, lax-jointedness was associated with becoming a good athlete. At the same time, however, when the football injuries were counted up, it was found that the lax-jointed football players had *more* than their share of injuries when compared to their normal teammates. So, here again, lax-jointedness indicates a predisposition to injuries such as sprains. A similar study of English ballet dancers came to much the same conclusion: dancers, when compared to nurses, tended to display a laxity in all of their joints, including those that were not specifically stretched by the dancing training process. This suggested that lax-jointedness is one of the things that make a good dancer rather than that dancing causes the joints to become lax.

However, most of the rheumatic problems of lax-jointedness occur in later life, if at all. People with over-supple feet tend to develop fallen arches which become painful; in others the knees, which may to some extent bend back to front, develop premature osteoarthritis (Chapter 6); in the hands, the supple-jointed person, when young, may be able to get his thumb to bend back so far that he can let it lie along the forearm, but because of this, when he gets older, the same thumb joint may become prematurely damaged and stiff.

The extreme forms of lax-jointedness are seen in some circus contortionists, but these people usually also have exceptional muscle strength which helps to protect their joints.

9

Rheumatism in Children

The legend referred to at the beginning of the first chapter states that it was the graceful antelope who decided to doom man the hunter with the curse of rheumatism in his joints. But according to the legend, the antelope relented because of the beauty of man's children and modified the curse so that it should only affect man in adult life.

But children *do* get rheumatism. It is far less common than in adults and, fortunately, it does not often progress to serious crippling arthritis. But, nevertheless, there are at least 250,000 children in the United States who do have juvenile rheumatoid arthritis. The ratio of children who do suffer from a rheumatic attack of any kind is tiny in comparison to those who don't — if roughly one word in this chapter equals the child sufferer then all the other words represent the healthy children. But if you've had any experience of children you will know that the child who complains at one time or another of rheumatic pains is not nearly so rare. Mild, temporary, and unimportant aches and pains are so common that a special term — growing pains — has developed to embrace them all. One good way of distinguishing the serious from the unimportant types of rheumatism is by looking for swelling of the joints. If a child complains of an arm, a leg, or a joint that is swollen, it is usually important. If the child complains of pain in the arm or leg but there is no swelling, it may be important but usually it is not.

This chapter will deal with:

1. Mild, pretended, and psychological rheumatism in children

2. The two most well-known rheumatic conditions in children — rheumatic fever and Still's disease

3. The rarer causes of arthritis in children, including the attacks associated

257

with certain diseases

ACHES AND PAINS

Growing Pains

Why do some children get growing pains? Quite often the explanation is simply that the child is seeking attention. "Mummy, I can't get to sleep because my feet hurt" often means the same as "I can't get to sleep; may I have a glass of water?" Or "Mummy, will you read me a story?" Parents are naturally concerned about their children's health and many children soon learn that complaints about an arm or a leg hurting elicit more attention than other tried devices.

Sometimes the child is just copying the mother. The mother who says, "I must put my legs up, my feet are killing me" is associating the two ideas of lying down and having painful feet. Children are great mimics and they try out this idea. Their feet hurt too when they lie down. If this makes their mother concerned and sympathetic, they are more likely to do it again. And again and again. Until in desperation, the mother takes her child to a doctor.

If such complaints are recognized as just the equivalent of asking for a bedtime story, then the wise mother will read a bedtime story, not forgetting of course to look at the so-called painful limb to reassure the child and herself that there is nothing wrong. Handled this way, the child seldom complains for very long.

Handled some other way, the situation may build up until both mother and child are convinced of the onset of some terrible disease. The contrast of the doctor not being able to find anything wrong may even increase the mother's worry. This type of situation is very common, particularly where there are sensitive and imaginative children and a parent who is prone to worrying. Girls seem more liable to become affected than boys, but it is usually nothing more than a phase in the child's development occurring between the ages of two and ten. Given tact and patience, the growing pains disappear in the same inexplicable way they started. Growing pains are not, strictly speaking, a disease but many doctors use the term because of the lack of any other name.

The fact that the joints are not swollen is a good indication that nothing serious is amiss. But occasionally the doctor may decide to prove that the complaints are nothing more than growing pains by asking for X-rays and blood tests. This helps to rule out any possibility of a serious disease since in growing pains there are no changes on the X-ray and the blood tests are normal. The danger here is in the effect this may have on the child. He or she may be convinced that because a fuss is being made (X-rays and a prick in the arm), something *must* be wrong. The wisest way for the doctor to handle this is to reassure the mother and child of his belief in the fact that nothing is wrong and explain that the tests are just routine.

Cold-Sensitive Pain

Another form of trivial rheumatism of which children often complain is pain in the feet and ankles during cold weather. This tends to affect boys more than girls. In a typical situation, a boy about ten or eleven years old stands around for a long time watching a football match in cold, wet shoes; even once he is home and is wearing dry shoes and socks, his feet may continue to ache for several hours. This, of course, isn't true arthritis, it is merely cold-induced pain. For example, if you take a block of ice and hold it tightly in one hand for several minutes, your hand not only feels cold, it also hurts. If you hold the ice longer, the pain becomes more and more severe and spreads up the arm until it is even felt in the chest. The pain, in this experiment, is due to the ice literally chilling the bones inside the hand. Bones and other structures below the skin cannot feel cold, they can only feel pain.

People vary in their susceptibility to cold-induced pain. Some will notice little or no pain when they hold the ice cube. Similarly, in children, some feel pain whenever their legs are chilled, while others hardly ever have this problem.

The answer, of course, is to avoid any situation that creates the aching, to wear warm socks and waterproof shoes. However, if the feet do become chilled, a hot soak in a bath or a hot water bottle in the bed will soon ease the aching.

Psychological or Psychosomatic Pains

Children occasionally complain of pain in their limbs as an expression of personal or family tension. This could arise from a feeling of insecurity, which some children have if their parents are arguing continuously. The doctor cannot do anything in this sort of situation; it is up to the parents to provide a peaceful home or temporarily send the child away. Or it could be because the child has nightmares, or because he is bullied at school. Any number of events or circumstances could lead him to complain of pains rather than about the real cause of his worry. If the situation with regard to school bullying or nightmares is recognized, it may be possible to change it and stop the complaint.

These are some of the less important sorts of childhood rheumatism. The next section deals with the more serious kinds.

RHEUMATIC FEVER

The disappearance of rheumatic fever in affluent countries has been one of the great medical victories of the last half-century. Around 1900, something like half of all the children admitted to the medical wards of the Hospital for Sick Children in London were suffering from rheumatic fever and its complications. The Medical Research Council Rheumatism Unit at Taplow, England, was originally set up in 1945 specifically to deal with children suffering from severe rheumatic fever. Recently they have been able to state confidently that "Rheumatic fever is now a rare and comparatively mild disease," and they are now concentrating their work on other forms of rheumatism in children. Unfortunately, this statement does not apply in less affluent countries such as Egypt, Mexico, and India, where even today the wards are full of children suffering from severe rheumatism with heart disease.

The Cause of Rheumatic Fever . . .

Rheumatic fever is one of the few rheumatic diseases for which the cause is known. It always follows an infection of the throat with a special kind of microorganism, the hemolytic streptococcus, producing what is commonly known as a strep throat. Having a strep throat does not necessarily mean that the child will get rheumatic fever — even in the bad old days no more than 3 percent of strep throats were followed by rheumatic fever. Today thousands of children have strep throats without a single instance of rheumatic fever becoming apparent. But occasional patients with rheumatic fever do turn up, and without exception they have evidence in their blood of having previously had streptococcal infection of the throat.

. . . And of its Disappearance

The disappearance of rheumatic fever may have been partly due to the availability of antibiotics such as penicillin. This has made possible prompt treatment of streptococcal infection of the throat and elimination of the cause. But this doesn't seem to be the whole answer, and many scientists think that the general improvement in living standards has in some way increased our resistance. Others think that the organism itself has become less virulent.

What Happens in Rheumatic Fever

Some seven to fourteen days after the throat infection the child who is going to get an attack of rheumatic fever becomes feverish and often looks pale and ill. One or more of the joints will swell and become painful. Often one joint swells when another one has just begun to improve; this condition is aptly named

265

migratory arthritis. This arthritis and fever make it imperative to keep the child in bed. Other signs of an attack include the development of small nodules (which are about the size of a grain of wheat) on the elbows or knuckles, and a peculiar rash on the arms and trunk.

Heart Involvement

There is a saying that rheumatic fever "licks the joints and bites the heart." Certainly, the greatest threat in rheumatic fever is the possibility of involvement of the heart. This takes the form of an inflammation of the heart's three coats, the pericardium or outer coat, the myocardium or muscle, and the endocardium or lining.

Pericarditis Inflammation of the outer coat of the heart may produce pain, usually felt in the front of the chest, spreading to the left shoulder. Breathing intensifies the pain, and children with this condition sometimes become very short of breath.

Myocarditis Inflammation of the heart muscle can occur. One result is the development of an irregular pulse and other changes which can be picked up on the electrocardiogram.

Endocarditis Inflammation of the lining of the heart can involve the valves, which may stretch and become inefficient. Years later, often after many attacks, the valves become thick and fail to open and close properly. This interferes with the heart's efficiency as a pump, and if it is severe may lead to long-term disability from breathlessness.

St. Vitus' Dance

One occasional accompaniment of rheumatic fever is chorea or St. Vitus' dance. This consists of involuntary movements and twitches, often starting in one side of the body. Because of this, the child appears clumsy and frequently drops things. And to make it worse, it is not unusual for children with this

267

condition to find themselves being punished for breaking the crockery while doing the dishes. Although it may persist for a long time, it is not often serious and never leaves permanent changes.

Prevention

Most diseases of children, such as mumps, are the sort that confer immunity, so that once the child has had one attack, he becomes immune and will never develop another. But with rheumatic fever the situation is quite different. Once he has had one attack he is more liable to have another. To prevent recurrences a child may be given penicillin tablets daily or a monthly injection of a long-acting penicillin that will stop any fresh streptococcal sore throat.

If the heart has been involved in the child's first attack, then it is almost certain that there will be heart involvement in any recurrent attacks. But if he escaped it in the first attack he will escape it in further attacks. For this reason many doctors do not insist on long-term prevention of rheumatic fever in children who have never had any heart involvement. But they will usually insist that every new sore throat be treated promptly with penicillin or some other antibiotic to make sure that the organism doesn't get a fresh foothold.

The question of how long prevention should go on has no certain answer. Most authorities argue that children with rheumatic heart disease should continue taking penicillin for at least five years after the last attack or until they leave school — whichever is the longer.

Rheumatic Heart Disease

In those rare instances where a child has rheumatic fever and is left with rheumatic heart disease, the question arises "Can anything be done?" Apart from preventing recurrences of rheumatic fever to lessen the chances of making the rheumatic heart trouble worse, it is also possible today to correct some of the damage surgically.

The commonest valve lesion, mitral stenosis — a narrowing of the mitral valve — is fairly easily corrected surgically. The next most frequent, mitral incompetence, is a widening of the valve base so that blood refluxes at each stroke of the heart beat. It can also be treated but is a little more difficult. The operation involves replacing the natural valve with an artificial one. Even more difficult, but now possible, is the operation to correct damage to the aortic valve. In some patients surgeons have successfully corrected both the mitral and the aortic valves in one operation.

One problem which should be mentioned here is that when teeth are extracted or filled, many of the bacterial organisms that normally live in the mouth are liberated into the blood stream for a short period. This infection is likely to settle in the heart valves damaged by rheumatic fever and could therefore be serious. For this reason, anyone with rheumatic heart disease should receive an antibiotic such as penicillin at the time of any dental treatment.

The Tonsils and Rheumatic Fever

There is no evidence that removing the tonsils will make any difference to the rheumatism caused by strep throats. But in fact some sufferers need to have their tonsils removed purely because of a tendency to repeated infection or the formation of abscesses.

STILL'S DISEASE (JUVENILE RHEUMATOID ARTHRITIS)

George Frederick Still was the first man to understand that there is a chronic form of arthritis in children which is not just a long-lasting variety of rheumatic fever. He was a physician at the Hospital for Sick Children in London, and in his time this particular disease — now named after him — was much less common than rheumatic fever. It is still rare, though it now probably seems more frequent because rheumatic fever has become so scarce.

Current theories about Still's disease

suggest that it is usually a juvenile form of rheumatoid arthritis (see Chapter 4). Only six in every ten thousand schoolchildren get some form of Still's disease, and in many of these cases it is only mild and fleeting. Eighty percent recover completely, being left with minor changes that can only be detected by experts or by the use of X-rays; of those who develop trouble in adult life, some have a condition that is indistinguishable from rheumatoid arthritis, and others develop a condition that resembles ankylosing spondylitis (see Chapter 2).

What is Still's Disease?

There are three main types of Still's disease:
1. In one kind there is a swelling in one or two of the main joints. The knees and wrists in particular are affected. After a period of time — often long — the swelling clears up. The knee usually recovers completely but the wrist tends to stiffen up as it heals, so that it won't move through its normal range.

2. Another common kind is similar to adult rheumatoid arthritis. The hands and feet are affected: the small joints of the fingers, toes, wrists, and ankles swell up, and, to some extent, the other larger joints may be troublesome as well. In the most severe cases of this variety, the neck, shoulders, and hips are involved, which means that the children may become severely crippled.

3. The third type of Still's disease starts as a persistent fever and illness in which there is often initially no joint trouble at all. It is only after some time that the joint disease develops, and even then it is mild, and it is the fever and general illness that dominate the picture.

These three main kinds of Still's disease are not always so well defined in practice. There are also all sorts of intermediate varieties. But although it is possible that one kind will develop into another type of Still's disease, usually this does not happen.

It is important to stress that Still's disease is not just arthritis of the joints. Many other parts of the body can be affected.

The skin may show a peculiar sort of rash in the form of little red blotches present in the morning over the trunk and limbs, often disappearing in the afternoon. The doctor who always makes his visits after lunch may miss it. Other children develop swelling of the lymph nodes in the neck and in the armpit. Some become anemic. A few develop inflammation around the outer coat of the heart — pericarditis — similar to that which may occur in rheumatic fever, but not involving the lining and the valves of the heart.

Perhaps the most alarming complication is when the eyes become involved; inflammation of the iris may occasionally lead to blindness. This inflammation can occur in the eyes of children only mildly affected by arthritis. As the early eye symptoms can be minimal, and young children may not appreciate them and make them known, a careful watch must be kept for the earliest signs of this complication, as with proper treatment, blindness can usually be prevented.

Who Is Affected and Why?

Nobody really knows what causes Still's disease. There is some evidence to imply that a tendency to get this condition is inherited. Boys with Still's disease tend to have more relatives with ankylosing spondylitis than chance would suggest. In twin studies, when one twin is affected, both members of identical twin pairs are more frequently affected than is the case with non-identical twin pairs. But inheritance does not provide us with the complete explanation. The truth is that we just do not know what the cause or causes are, or even if it is one single condition or several slightly different ones.

Still's disease can start early in life: the youngest recorded case is in a baby of nine months. Girls are more frequently affected than boys, the ratio being about 3:1. Another feature is the broad variety of its victims; Still's disease is no respecter of the rich or the poor; both seem equally vulnerable. Nothing in the way of food that is eaten, exposure to damp, exercise, or other illness seems particularly liable to bring it on.

Still's Disease and Stunted Growth

The fact that children are still growing when they contract what is otherwise an adult disease radically affects the situation. A sick child usually fails to grow properly and a chronically sick child may end up shorter than his normal brothers and sisters. Also, the age of puberty will arrive later for the sick child.

The situation with Still's disease is even more pronounced: when a joint is badly inflamed the growing part of the bone — which is near the joint — may be affected. At first, it may be stimulated so that the bone grows faster than normal. But subsequently it is often damaged so that it fails to grow. This can produce results in which one arm or leg is shorter than the other, or one toe is shorter than the rest.

In the past the problem was increased because cortisone and its derivatives, prednisone and many other similar drugs (see Chapter 4), which are often given for the relief of pain and inflammation in Still's disease, specifically act to stop growth. The dilemma for the doctor was, should the child be given other, weaker tablets which might not give such good pain relief but which would allow the child to grow more or less normally? Happily, this question is resolved today, as it is now possible to use these drugs to provide good relief of pain and inflammation, without the penalty of stunting, in all but the most difficult instances.

Treatment of Still's Disease

Drugs Drug treatment is similar to that given for adult rheumatoid arthritis. There are two classes of treatment.

1. There are the quick-acting tablets that relieve pain and inflammation. The simplest of these is aspirin, and the most powerful is cortisone or its derivatives.

2. The second class of treatment is concerned with long-term suppression of the illness. Gold injections and immuno-suppressive drugs are among those that

can be given.

Children with severe disease may need a drug of each class. However, and this point needs to be stressed, the treatment of Still's disease does not just come out of a bottle of pills. Many other things are vitally important:

Rest and exercise It is important that children with Still's disease have exactly the right amount of rest. It needs to be prescribed just like medicine — too much is as bad for them as too little. Joints that are becoming bent may need splints or, if this fails, an operation to get them straight. Complications like anemia may need to be tackled so as to improve the child's general resistance to disease. A most important kind of physical therapy is probably the hot pool, where a physical therapist may teach the child to keep his joints free and his muscles strong. The children are delighted to have the chance of moving joints in warm water which, if moved on dry land, might be painful. In general, children need much less rest than adults and are much better when kept active, even if they have a fever and their joints are swollen. But how much rest and exercise and how much splinting are necessary for each individual child are matters to be decided by an expert.

Hospitalization and education Child psychologists urge that, if at all possible, a sick child should be nursed at home. If this is not possible, he should be admitted to a hospital near enough to home to allow the family to visit frequently. But when the disease is severe and prolonged, this is not the only consideration. A crippled child may have to work with his head rather than with his hands and it is vitally important that he go to a hospital that has a school so that he can continue his education. In Britain, for example, many children are treated at the special unit for Juvenile Rheumatism at Taplow, near London. There are several centers in the United States that specialize in treating children with arthritis and rheumatism, among them centers in Worcester (Massachusetts), Houston, Los Angeles, and New York.

Surgery It is occasionally necessary to operate on joints that have been severely damaged by Still's disease. The most common operations are on the hips, knees, and wrists to prevent stiffening or contractions. Artficial hips have now been successfully put into children and a great deal can be done by surgeons to correct bad positions of the knees and wrists. But such operations are rarely needed these days when splints and exercise can help prevent deformity. Children are in many ways much tougher than adults. They have a remarkable ability to recover from what often seem impossible circumstances, including being affected by a devastating disease.

The future Most children with Still's disease grow up perfectly normal. They may end up being rather shorter than their school fellows but their intelligence is not affected. They live normal lives, get married, and have children. Since there is no evidence that the condition is directly inherited, there is no need for them to worry about passing it on to their children.

RARER CAUSES OF ARTHRITIS IN CHILDREN

There are a large number of rarer causes of arthritis and joint disease in children and only a few of them will be considered here. It is often difficult to distinguish one from another and a skilled specialist has to be called in to give the diagnosis.

The same problem sometimes exists in sorting out rheumatic illnesses from some of the commoner childhood diseases. Any child who is developing a feverish illness is liable to get aches and pains in the back and limbs, especially when his temperature is going up. The child will usually look ill, may vomit, shiver, and have a hot forehead even if the hands and feet look pale and feel cold. This sort of aching is particularly common before the onset of measles and German measles. But it may precede any of the childhood fevers such as mumps and chickenpox. The pains often arrive several days before the rash appears (in measles or chickenpox) or before the glands swell (in mumps). Except in an epidemic, even the doctor may find it difficult to say what illness the child is developing in this early stage of fever and aches and pains in the limbs.

German Measles

In some epidemics of German measles (rubella) those affected develop a true arthritis and not just the aches and pains of a fever. Some of the larger joints in the body swell and become painful. The same arthritis can also occur in adults, usually young women, and then it is sometimes confused with the onset of rheumatoid arthritis. This arthritis may last for several weeks or even a month or two, but it practically always seems to clear up. It is therefore a relatively trivial problem.

Meningitis

A word of warning is needed. If the aches and pains are accompanied by pains in the back and neck, and particularly if the neck is so stiff that the child cannot bring his head forward on to his chest, it may be due to an infection of the outer lining of the brain. In meningitis (cerebrospinal fever) and in poliomyelitis (infantile paralysis), headache and stiff neck are common early in the illness. In poliomyelitis this is often accompanied by quite severe pains in one or another of the limbs.

Erythema Nodosum

Another childhood skin condition that is sometimes associated with a type of arthritis is erythema nodosum. This strange-sounding name refers to a painful blotchy rash that appears on the shins in the form of reddish lumpy swellings. These are tender to touch and eventually show deep bruising. In itself this is a trivial condition and the arthritis that accompanies it is usually transient, but the doctor will want to investigate it thoroughly as it is occasionally associated with other more serious internal disease.

Psoriasis

Chapter 5 described in some detail the different ways in which psoriasis can be associated with arthritis in adults. The first attack of psoriasis, which appears as a persistent rash consisting of angry red patches covered with silvery scales, often occurs in childhood. When it does, there is about a 5 percent chance that it will be accompanied by a form of arthritis similar to Still's disease. The problems and treatment are much the same as those of Still's disease.

Hemophilia

It is common knowledge that hemophilia is a bleeding disease, but the fact that it is also a disease of the joints is not so widely known. It is one of the few conditions that is definitely inherited, and as such it has a royal history.

Descendants of Queen Victoria married into the Russian royal family and transmitted the disease there. Crown Prince Alexei, heir to the Czar of Russia during the First World War, was subject to disastrous episodes of bleeding into his joints. Because of this, as many old pictures show, he was carried around on the shoulders of a sailor in the Czar's Navy. The monk Rasputin claimed to be able to stop the bleeding and because of this exercised an extraordinary influence over the boy's mother, the Czarina Alexandra.

Hemophilia only affects boys, but women can transmit the disease to their sons. A daughter of a hemophiliac has a 50 percent chance of becoming a carrier.

Characteristically, boys who are affected will bleed for a long time even after mild wounds. Some boy babies have died from continuous bleeding after circumcision. In other patients it is difficult to stop the bleeding after a tooth has been extracted. But while mild cases just show prolonged bleeding, the more severely affected bleed under the skin into the muscles or joints. This can cause deformity and crippling.

It is now possible to prevent joint damage in patients with hemophilia. Although hemophilia cannot be cured, it can be treated. If normal blood is separated into plasma and red cells and the plasma is put in a cold refrigerator under certain conditions, some solid material settles out of it and is known as cryoprecipitate. It contains the particular substances that are deficient in hemophiliac boys. If cryoprecipitate is given promptly to the boy, it will stop the bleeding immediately.

It is therefore most important for the family with a hemophiliac child to live near one of the major hemophilia centers. The parents of such children are often given the privilege of calling the ambulance themselves to take the child directly to the center if bleeding is suspected, without first trying to get hold of the family doctor. The more practical and intelligent parents can be taught to give an intravenous injection of cryoprecipitate. This can be kept for emergencies in the family refrigerator. A useful temporary measure, which can also be kept in the refrigerator, is the instant cold pack, a plastic bag full of a material that will not freeze. When this is placed over a joint that has been subjected to bleeding it can relieve pain and will probably stop the bleeding until other help arrives.

Today the greatest danger to the hemophiliac is the car accident. Ironically, once joint damage has occurred, the sufferers are even more dependent than the rest of us on car transport, but even a minor accident may be dangerous for a hemophiliac. Auto accident statistics are daunting for us all — the probability of one car accident for every 50,000 miles driven by the average motorist in the United States — but for the hemophiliac they are frightening and alarming. As a precaution, all hemophiliacs should carry a special identity card which gives their disease and blood group in case they need an emergency transfusion.

Vitamin Deficiencies

Scurvy develops in babies when there is a deficiency of vitamin C in the diet. This may occur if the child has been kept on artificial milk feedings for too long without being given orange juice or any other source of vitamin C. As a result, there is a tendency for bleeding in and around the joints. This is very painful, but luckily the condition is usually quite apparent to a skilled pediatrician.

Rickets is another vitamin deficiency disease that causes trouble to joints. In this case it is due to a deficiency of vitamin D, the sunshine vitamin. Such children tend to be stunted, their arms and legs grow bent, and their joints may feel painful. Curing rickets is usually straightforward, but a few children may need enormous doses of vitamin D, as they are resistant to it. However, too much vitamin D can also be bad, and blood tests are needed to check that the right dose is being used.

Bone Diseases

Many bone diseases in children initially appear to be a form of rheumatism. The most serious is an infection of the bone — osteomyelitis. If the infection is located near the joint, the child will often complain of pain in the joint. It is usually very painful and causes the child to become generally ill and have a fever. Diagnosis can be difficult, as X-rays do not show any changes until late in the diease. It may be necessary to prescribe antibiotic treatment without having any positive proof of the existence of infection.

Leukemia

Leukemia in children sometimes presents itself as a form of rheumatism. This is because the bone marrow near the joints may become involved and thus irritate the joints. The joint may swell, and, of course, the bones nearby will become painful. Important medical advances have been made, making it possible to prolong the lives of children who are affected by leukemia and in relieving much of their suffering.

PREVENTING ARTHRITIS AND RHEUMATISM IN ADULT LIFE

Some children are born with congenital dislocation of the hip. The hip is not correctly positioned in its socket. If they are allowed to walk like this, they will develop lifelong deformities and a peculiar waddling gait. Today pediatricians examine newborn babies for dislocation of the hip; if this is detected, the position of the hip can be corrected and the child nursed in a special splint until the hip stays in its socket in a normal manner.

Another condition which, if treated when the patient is young, need not cause permanent damage is Legg-Perthe's disease. This is a disease of adolescent children in which the growing part of the bone near the hip joint becomes damaged. It usually occurs in rather overweight children. They complain of pain in the groin and begin to limp. If treated early, the condition may settle down without any serious after-effects; but if neglected, the hip joint may be permanently damaged so that serious trouble arises in later life.

10

Painful Feet

The structure of the human foot, bone for bone and joint for joint, is very similar to the human hand. But there the resemblance ends. We cannot possibly do the same things with the feet as with the hands, or vice versa. For example, we cannot grasp objects or play the piano with our toes, neither can the hands bear the weight of the body for more than a few minutes. We marvel at the weightlifter who is able to use his hands to lift several times his own body weight above his head for a few seconds. We forget that the same man's feet also have to carry the additional amount of weight plus the weight of his body. Moreover the feet — which are constructed in the same way as the hand — must carry the body weight all day and every day.

The hand is on show; gloves are worn only for protection against hard work or weather. The foot is usually hidden; coverings of socks, stockings and shoes prevent exposure. The hand is free to move in any direction; the foot is cramped in its containers. Rings are worn to accentuate the delicate apearance of the female hand; the foot is often considered to be unattractive, dirty, and smelly. Consequently, more concern is given to the shoe that covers the foot than to the foot inside the shoe. Far too many people, particularly young women, buy shoes primarily to be fashionable and do not worry about whether they actually fit. It is inevitable that such people will be afflicted later on by a number of unnecessary and often uncomfortable troubles in their feet. These may have nothing to do with rheumatism, but if rheumatism or arthritis does develop in the feet, it is not just a question of discomfort but of serious, painful, and crippling deformity. The possibility should not be dismissed as unlikely:

arthritis is the greatest cause of foot troubles. After all, there are over twenty joints in each foot and any one, or all of them, can be affected by arthritis.

THE ANATOMY OF THE FOOT

The Structure

One of the most important but least considered parts of the foot is the curious fibrous and fatty cushion that separates the sole from the bones. It is the structure of this that enables the foot to bear enormous pressures.

The soles of people who don't wear shoes become horny and thick until the skin is just like tough leather. In fact, to be accurate, it *is* tough leather. People who wear shoes have thinner soles but the skin is still very tough. Between this skin and the bony skeleton inside there is a sponge-like feltwork of fibers. The spaces between the fibers are filled in with soft fat which forms the cushions of the heel and under the joints at the base of the toes.

The bones of the feet are arranged in two so-called arches, the longitudinal and the transverse arch. The longitudinal arch describes the bones from the heel to the base of the toes. This supports the bones of the lower leg. The height of the arch varies enormously. It is possible to have either a high arch or a flat one which only appears while the person is standing on tip-toe — both are normal. It is also quite normal for toddlers to have very flat feet. The transverse arch refers to the bones at the front of the foot. The five bones at the base of the toes are arranged so that it is mainly the big toe joint that carries the

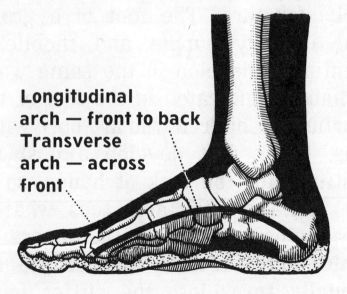

Longitudinal
arch — front to back
Transverse
arch — across
front

The two arches of the foot

weight, supported to some extent by the bones of the little toe joint. In between, the bones form an arch that is able to support weight in abnormal conditions, or when the foot is under strain as in jumping or running, but they do not normally do so.

The muscles, tendons, and ligaments are situated around the bones and allow for the springiness and suppleness of the foot.

The Development

A baby's foot is full of fat and without much structure. The foot of a growing child is very supple and mobile. Its potential to develop in the same way as the hand is indicated in the feet of those unfortunate children who are born without arms. Their feet develop almost as a substitute for the lack of hands, so that they can do with their toes what can normally be done only by the fingers. This supple and trainable foot of the child gradually turns into the stiffer foot of adult life which is unable to function in any way other than that for which it is always used — namely supporting the weight of the body.

Even in adult life, however, people's feet differ in the degree of stiffness or suppleness of the inside structures. This is often very significant. Two people may have exactly the same size and shape of foot at rest; but one person can have a rigid foot and so need a shoe that is an exact fit, whereas the other person may have a supple foot and can probably wear a shoe that is too small or the wrong shape, and feel little or no pain.

The Nerve Supply

The feet are second only to the hands in the richness of the nerve supply from the brain. This means that they are sensitive structures which, if damaged, are capable of giving rise to a great deal of pain. Even touching the skin can cause an unpleasant sensation — there are tales of a Chinese torture that consists of tickling the feet for several hours at a time. As in other parts of the body, the hard parts of the joints do not contain any pain nerve endings but the ligaments, tendons, and skin around the joints are rich in pain fibers. This is particularly true of the skin around the nails.

The nerves to the feet also control the extent of sweating of the foot. Again, the wide variation between people's sweating feet is quite normal. In a moist, sweaty foot the skin may become soggy and decompose. The process is in fact similar to the rotting of moist leaves in a compost heap and is brought about by germs. The structure of the skin changes and becomes softer — it can often be scraped off between the toes and around the nails. At the same time the decomposition produces the characteristic "cheesy" foot odors. Although the smell is an old problem, in modern days it is probably more severe. The reason for this is that such odors are more common in feet shod with impermeable shoes made of modern plastics than in feet shod in traditional leather which to some extent allows the foot to breathe.

The Blood Supply

The foot has a good blood supply carried by two main arteries, one coming down in front of the ankle and one behind the ankle bone on the inner side of the heel. In older people and in diabetics, this circulation often fails. It is possible for it to block completely, in which case there is considerable pain, and there may even be gangrene due to loss of the blood supply. Diabetes with loss of blood supply is one of the main causes of leg amputation. Most of these patients will have suffered severe foot pain before the decision is finally made to amputate. This pain is often initially attributed to rheumatism.

SHOES AND FOOT DEFORMITY

Barefoot in the Park

Shoes cause more foot problems than anything else, and faulty shoes are especially to blame. If we didn't wear shoes, there would probably be about 90 percent fewer foot troubles than are suffered today. But if we did go around barefoot there would no doubt be pain from other sources: frostbite in cold climates; cuts from thorns and sharp stones; bites from insects and snakes; infestation in tropical countries from certain sorts of parasitic worms. Ideally, the child should grow up in an always equable climate and do nothing but run around in bare feet on a grass lawn all day. He would presumably grow up without any foot deformities at all. But this idyllic situation just does not exist. We have to wear shoes to protect our feet and to that extent we have to accept that a certain number of foot deformities are likely to be with us however much we attempt to avoid them.

Aching Feet — A Common Problem?

May Clarke, in a sample survey of the feet of British people in 1969, estimated that at least 50 percent, and possibly 80 percent, of the people in that country had something the matter with their feet. Similar findings would occur in any other relatively affluent, shoe-wearing country. Most of these disorders are relatively trivial, such as ingrown toenails, corns, athlete's foot, or minor bunions. But some are serious, particularly in older women. For them, foot deformities and nail problems constitute a major source of pain and disability. There are probably no more than two or three in every hundred women who have reached the age of eighty and still have normal feet. Arthritis of the feet is far less common but the intense problems that it causes are much greater. From various estimates it is possible to guess that about 2 percent of the adult population suffer from arthritis of the feet. At least nine out of every ten rheumatoid arthritics have trouble with their feet, whereas the hands are affected in only seven out of every ten.

Foot Development — From Dainty to Deformed

How do the perfect little feet of the baby become the rather unpleasant objects that support the weight of the adult? At what stage do deformities start and how can they be prevented? And once a deformity has developed, is it possible to re-straighten the foot?

The infant's foot until about the age of ten is a rapidly growing structure that is very soft and mobile. It is a mistake to view the baby's foot as a miniature adult foot, for it has a different shape. This means that the shape of a baby's shoe must not imitate the shape of an adult's shoe. It is particularly important for the child's shoe to have a straight inner border and be long enough to allow the toes to wriggle inside the toe cap. As the toddler grows, he may still crawl as much as he walks and his shoes will wear out as quickly on top as on the sole. From the age of four upward, boys are particularly hard on their shoes; few small boys can resist playing football in their best shoes.

This is, in fact, a blessing in disguise, since it means that the shoes wear out quickly and have to be replaced. Girls are often less fortunate; because they take longer to wear their shoes out, they tend to continue wearing the same shoes for longer periods. This means that the foot often outgrows the shoe and this is one of the reasons why girls get more foot deformities than boys.

The first foot deformities begin in infancy with the tucking-in of the little toe under the fourth toe. This is probably due to tight socks and shoes which, even if they don't seem too tight, nevertheless compress the toes. However, foot deformities at this age, and even up to the age of ten or more, are completely reversible provided that the child is taken out of the constriction of socks and shoes.

But after the age of ten, and particularly in the adolescent years for girls (between twelve and sixteen), shoe deformities tend to become permanent. Also, it is in this age range that girls are first prone to develop the sort of deformities that plague them throughout their adult life. It is a critical time; their feet may grow by as much as half an inch in six months, but because children's feet are relatively insensitive they may wear tight shoes without complaint.

New shoes are expensive but so are old ones — in a different way. If the toes are cramped together during the vital finishing stage of the development of the foot, they are then molded crooked for life. It is at this stage that the bunions form, or the small toes become packed together and sooner or later become painful. The survey of schoolchildren's feet conducted by Dr. Catherine Hollman found that over half of all children had a bunion by the age of fifteen and that girls were affected three times as often as boys.

In order to prevent this, barefoot activities should be encouraged as often as possible on the beach or in the fields, or even in the streets, and especially in the home. Whenever there is no danger to feet from cold weather, thorns, or stones children should be encouraged to do without shoes and in the summer to wear open-toed sandals. Tight socks are a special hazard. A wool sock that has shrunk, a nylon stretch sock, or just simply a cotton sock that has been outgrown — any of these can bend the little toe against the others and sometimes right under or over the fourth toe. It is particularly important not to try and make shoes last too long at the stage when the child's foot is growing rapidly. For this reason, cheap shoes are often better than expensive ones since the temptation to make them last is not so great.

The worst offender for deforming girls' feet is the type of shoe that has a very tight, rather pointed toe cap, no heel support, and stays on the foot only by the grip on the toes. This necessarily packs the toes together. Young girls, already fashion-conscious but unfortunately not health-conscious, only too readily try to force their feet into shoes that they regard as elegant. As a result, their feet become inelegant.

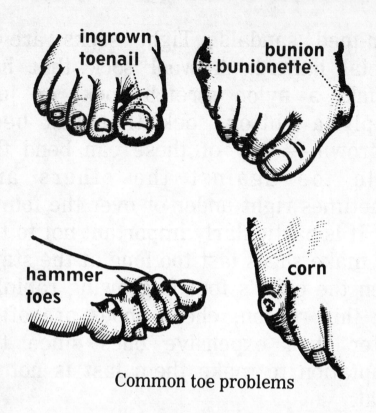

ingrown
toenail

bunion
bunionette

hammer
toes

corn

Common toe problems

Deformities in the Growing Foot

There is a long list of deformities caused by badly fitting shoes worn by growing children. First the nails suffer. Ingrown toenails are caused by pressure across the big toe and are often accompanied by deformities of other toenails. The joints of the big toe suffer with the development of a bunion that doctors call hallux valgus. The other toes develop a hammer toe deformity. The fifth toe is often pushed across to form a bunionette. The abnormal shape of the foot may mean that pressures develop between the skin and the shoe, causing corns. Other pressures on the foot may cause an exaggeration or loss of the normal springy arches of the foot, again with the later development of pain.

The Ideal Shoe

Shoes that are suitable for children will not compress the toes and will leave room for toe action. They will have a straight inner border so that the big toe can lie in

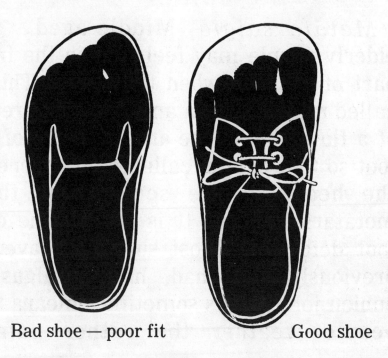

Bad shoe — poor fit   Good shoe

line with the inner side of the foot. They will clasp the heel reasonably firmly from side to side, and they will have something across the top, usually lacing, that will prevent the foot from sliding forward in the shoe during walking or running. They will have a heel that is about half an inch above the level of the sole and large enough to spread the weight of the body over a wide area.

PAIN IN THE FOOT

Pain in the Front Part of the Foot

Metatarsalgia Middle-aged and elderly people may feel pain in the front part of the foot when they walk. This is called metatarsalgia and is a direct result of a flattening of the anterior arch of the foot so that painful calluses form beneath the heads of the second and third metatarsal bones. It is seldom the only foot deformity. Most sufferers have, or previously have had, hallux valgus or bunion joints. This sometimes means that people weather the rather painful operation to have a hallux valgus removed, and are then disappointed to find that their feet are still in pain. This is because most operations for hallux valgus help to destroy the anterior arch of the foot, so that more weight is placed on the other bones. And if the vital fibro-fatty cushion is not very thick under these other bones, pain will result.

Morton's metatarsalgia A special kind of metatarsalgia is called Morton's metatarsalgia. In this condition one of the nerves to the toes gets nipped when it passes down in the cleft between the bones at the base of the toes. This is usually between the second and third toes. It can, of course, be extremely painful and is often associated with numbness of the skin on the sides of the toes. Eventually the painful nerve develops a little swelling called a neuroma which may need to be removed by an operation in order to relieve the pain.

March fracture Another painful condition in the forefoot is march fracture. This refers to a fracture in one of the metatarsal bones. It occurs for no obvious reason and can happen in healthy young men as well as in older patients who have some form of generalized weakness of their bones. The pain is acute and the condition is often misdiagnosed as arthritis, but an X-ray will immediately pinpoint the trouble.

Frieberg's disease Frieberg's disease is a curious degeneration of part of the bone at the base of the second toe in children's feet. The onset of this condition is thought to occur after there has been some local damage. Again, the diagnosis can easily be made by X-ray but the condition is not treatable except for protecting the foot until the discomfort disappears. Fortunately, most cases become painless although they may lead to some deformity of the joint.

Pain in the Middle Part of the Foot

Flat feet Flat feet are neither necessarily abnormal nor painful. The majority of flat feet in children are probably harmless and don't need treating. Very often such a child has a very mobile foot and the flat appearance only occurs when they are standing — as soon as they begin to walk, run, or jump, the flat foot disappears. The appearance of a flat foot is sometimes due to a child having a short Achilles tendon at the back of the heel. The child (usually a girl) can only stand barefoot if she lets the ankles fall inward. But few children have trouble in later life because their feet were flat as children. Indeed, several of them have ultimately become famous runners.

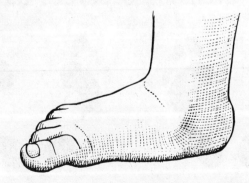

The normal flat foot in children

Some people, both young and old, do have pain caused by flat feet. The pain may be felt in the feet, ankles, and knees. Some corrections of the shoes may be necessary.

High arched feet The opposite of flat foot is an arch that is very high — called pes cavus by doctors. A person with pes cavus leaves a footprint that consists only of an unjoined print of the heel and the front of the foot. Often such a foot is only one end of the continuum of a normal foot. However, it may be associated with a hammer toe deformity and later with pressure sores forming on the top of the clawed toes. There may also be problems from pressure beneath the toe joints since they are taking all the weight. Sometimes this high arch is so severe as to be a

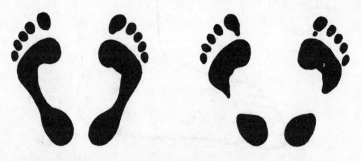

Prints from normal and high arched feet

312

deformity of the foot and it may result from diseases of the nerves which have caused a weakness or a contracture of the muscles to the foot. Poliomyelitis is one such cause.

Pain in the Back of the Foot

There are only two conditions that commonly arise in the back of the foot — plantar fasciitis and calcaneal bursitis.

Plantar fasciitis Plantar fasciitis means inflammation of the strong flat ligament, the plantar fascia, that runs from the heel bone to the toe bones along the sole of the foot. If you can imagine the foot as a bow, then this ligament acts like the string keeping it tight and maintaining the arch. The place where the fascia joins the bone at the heel, that is the enthesis,* often becomes strained and therefore painful. This condition is seen more often in men than in women and is sometimes a part of the abnormalities that accompany

* See Chapter 8 for a description of the enthesis.

313

various forms of arthritis.

The treatment of this can be quite difficult. Some patients respond quite well to putting a large ring-shaped pad made of thick felt inside the heel. The hole in the ring corresponds to the tender area. By using this, all the pressure is taken off the painful area that it can heal. Sometimes the tender spot can be injected with hydrocortisone. On other occasions anti-inflammatory medication is prescribed.

Calcaneal Bursitis The other part of the heel that quite frequently hurts is the area at the back where the strong Achilles tendon is attached. Again, this can develop as part of a generalized arthritis but it often occurs on its own. Suitable padding and injection treatment will usually relieve the pain to a reasonable extent. It is called calcaneal bursitis since it seems primarily to affect the little bursa or cushion that prevents the Achilles tendon and the back of the heel from rubbing.

There are various other, not so common, causes of pain around the ankle.

For example, the strong tendons that transmit the forces of the muscles in the calf down to the foot and the toes all have to take a sharp turning around the ankle, and to do this they pass through smooth, slippery tunnels known as synovial sheaths. These sheaths can become inflamed and distended with fluid, often as part of a generalized arthritis.

THE FOOT IN OLD AGE

Old people are particularly liable to have trouble with their feet. The foot, just like other parts of the body, changes with age. The skin under the foot becomes thin and not so elastic. The ligaments inside the foot become stiff and the whole foot structure becomes relatively rigid. The nails, although they grow slowly, tend to thicken and become hard to cut. Shoe deformities, such as bunions, gradually tend to get worse with age until the foot as well as being stiffer is also a good deal wider. If a person had a wide foot when young, then it may become impossible to find ready-made shoes that will fit the even wider older foot. Add to this the difficulties in stooping down to cut toenails or clean the toes, together with poor eyesight resulting in problems in seeing what they are doing, and it is then easy to see why many old people have a major problem with their feet.

THE FOOT IN ARTHRITIS

It has already been mentioned earlier in this chapter that nine out of ten people with rheumatoid arthritis get involvement of the joints of the feet. The joints most frequently affected are those at the base of the toes. Initially, they swell up, causing the whole of the front of the foot to be both wider and thicker. A patient with rheumatoid arthritis usually needs to wear shoes that are at least two sizes wider and often one size longer in order to allow enough room for the swollen foot. As a result, many women who develop rheumatoid arthritis have drawers and cupboards full of shoes which they have bought hoping for comfort and which they can no longer wear.

At the back of the foot, the joint most frequently affected in arthritis is the joint beneath the ankle that allows the heel to twist inward and outward. If no treatment is given for this, the ankles appear to drop inward.

In later rheumatoid arthritis the structure of the joints at the base of the toes softens, causing characteristic deformities from the pressures of standing and of wearing shoes. Hallux valgus or a bunion may become very severe. The smaller toes can be partially or completely dislocated at the joints at the base of the toe. Arthritis may also attack the bone near the joint so that it becomes rough or sharp and digs into the skin from inside.

More significant, however, is that the important fibro-fatty cushion moves forward away from the weight-bearing area so that only relatively thin skin separates the damaged joints from the ground. This skin typically reacts by producing corns or calluses which are often painful. At the same time, other calluses form on the tips of the toe near

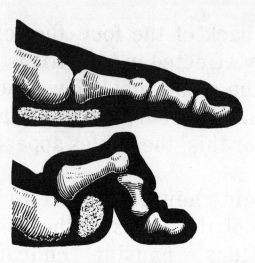

Dislocation of the toe joints and slipping forward of the protective pad

the nails, where the weight is being carried right on the point of the bone. In addition, more calluses are forming on top of the knuckles of the toes as they rub on the shoes. Because of the softening of the joints and the pressure of shoes, the smaller toes pack together in bizarre ways. Sometimes the little toe twists right underneath the others, sometimes it rides above them and the whole shape of the foot is distorted.

The later stages of arthritis in the back of the foot involve permanent deformity of the heel. Seen from the back of the foot it is quite clear how this upsets the way in which the weight of the body is carried down to the foot. Instead of the heel being in line with the leg, it is now displaced outward and the ankle inward. The weight of the body tends to aggravate the deformity. A special brace with a sling, known as a T-strap, may be necessary to prevent it becoming worse.

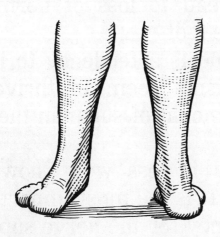

Bending in of the ankle and out of the heel

In the other forms of arthritis, those caused by ankylosing spondylitis, Reiter's syndrome, and the kind associated with psoriasis, the deformities of the foot are rather similar, although the pattern of involvement of the various parts of the foot tends to be a little different.

THE FOOT IN DIABETES

If arthritis is the biggest cause of foot troubles, it is closely followed by diabetes. Diabetes is complicated by three factors, all of which may affect the feet.

1. The first is a tendency to a hardening and eventually to blocking of arteries. This may lead to loss of normal blood supply to the foot.

2. The second is a tendency to infection. Microorganisms seem to thrive on the increased amount of sugar in the blood in diabetes.

3. The third is less well known but in many cases it is the most important. This is the tendency for the nerve supply to be interfered with so that the patient doesn't have the proper or appropriate sensations of pain. It is known as the diabetic neuropathic foot.

Because of the diabetes, there is interference in the conduction of the smallest nerve fibers which carry pain messages and control the sweating and circulation. This usually only occurs in severe diabetics but occasionally can be the first sign of this condition. Because of this failure to feel pain, in a bad case a patient may not realize that he is continuing to walk with a nail sticking through the sole of the shoe. Or the toes may be rubbing in an ill-fitting shoe. Sooner or later the skin breaks down, infection sets in, and a nasty ulcer, known as a penetrating ulcer, appears. If nothing is done and the patient continues to walk — as well he may because it doesn't hurt him — then the ulcer develops a spreading infection tunneling right into the structure of the foot. It may eventually almost destroy the foot.

Another problem is the development of fractures. A patient, not knowing that he has hurt himself, may continue to walk, and a small crack in the bone will progress to form an actual fracture that still elicits little or no pain.

This is not to say that diabetic patients with this problem don't get any pain in their feet at all. An ulcer that has started in a painless part of the foot may cause a great deal of pain when infection spreads to another part of the foot that is still capable of sending pain messages.

It follows that diabetics who have this complication need to exercise great care. They are advised to have a mirror placed on the floor in the bathroom and to inspect the soles of the feet regularly for any sores or raw areas; they must feel inside their shoes every day before putting them on to make sure that there is nothing in them that could cause abrasions. Their shoes must be soft and wide enough to give plenty of room, and if the shoe is to protect the foot, it must be kept dry. This means that diabetes is a special hazard for fishermen. They commonly wear rubber boots to keep their feet dry, but rubber boots which they can get into may be quite the wrong shape for their feet and may rapidly cause ulcers on the feet and deformities of the joints.

THE FOOT AND LEPROSY

The situation in diabetes is very similar to what happens to the feet in leprosy where infection of the nerves to the arms and legs causes loss of sensation. The deformities of the hands and feet in leprosy are directly due to this loss of the feeling of pain. Someone afflicted to leprosy can hold a hot pan or a cigarette so that it burns him without even being aware of it. This, in turn, causes the flesh, and eventually the bones, to ulcerate and disappear. Leprosy can now be cured, but in less affluent countries, with the rapid increase in population, the infection is spreading at a rate that outpaces attempts to cure it. Indeed, when one considers that leprosy can cause destruction of joints in fingers and feet, there is a good reason to make the startling statement that leprosy is probably now one of the most serious joint diseases in the world, but not, of course, in the United States.

TREATMENT

The Role of the Podiatrist

Modern podiatrists are highly trained. As with other professions, there are specialists among them; some concentrate on making beautifully molded foot appliances, others on providing special shoes, and others on the techniques of massage, manipulation, and remedial exercises for the foot. But most of general practice podiatry is concerned with the day-to-day care of the forefoot in older people — the cutting and cleaning of awkward toenails, the care and the dressings for corns and calluses, the provision of pads to help feet in pain from bunions or metatarsalgia. Most of these foot deformities are avoidable; they are the result of badly fitting shoes, weak foot muscles, or too much pressure due to obesity. They create an unfortunate burden on podiatrists, who are in short supply and are needed for other problems that are not yet preventable, such as the problems of arthritis in the feet or congenital deformity.

The main ways in which the podiatrist can help patients with arthritis of the feet are:

1. Ring pads. These take pressure off painful bony prominences by padding all around the area. The prominence goes through a hole in the middle. It is a common mistake for people trying to pad their own feet to put the padding on top of the prominence — this will only increase the pressure. The most suitable ring pads for bunion joints are made in the shape of a horseshoe, out of thick adhesive felt. Smaller ring pads for the knuckles of the toes are usually bought ready-made. Alternatively, the toes may be encased in animal wool which not only protects them but, because it is slippery, allows the sock or shoe to move over the painful area.

2. Toe pads. These are put between or under the toes to prop them into a better position. The painful calluses on the tips of clawed toes can often be corrected by a simple roll pad which the toes can grasp.

3. Metatarsal supports. Probably the most useful contribution of the podiatrist

concerns the various kinds of metatarsal support. These are pads designed to take the weight of the body off the painful joints at the base of the toes and transfer it farther back on to the soft parts of the foot. This is usually done by strapping specially made pads on to the foot. The disadvantage of this method is that the pads have to be removed for washing and then replaced — this can often be a long and complicated job.

In some patients, however, these pads are placed inside the shoe as a kind of insole. It is most important that the pad or metatarsal button is placed in exactly the right place. It is possible to have made special-shaped cork or composition insoles to meet each individual patient's requirements.

The problem about insoles or any other padding put in the shoe is that they are bulky and the shoe is often already too tight because of foot swelling. In fitting a shaped insole to persons with arthritis it is nearly always necessary to make sure that the patient has larger shoes. Certain podiatrists and footwear manufacturers carry a stock of shoes that are especially deeply lasted so as to make room not only for the foot but also for the insole. This is an ideal solution for people with mild foot deformity.

4. Valgus supports. These can be bought ready-made or in a form that can easily be molded into the shape that the individual requires, or they can be made individually out of molded plastic. Their job is to enable the area between the heel and the big toe — known in lay terms as the instep — to take some weight. They are needed only in secondary flat-foot which is due to disease of the joints in the foot. Unfortunately, they are also often supplied to young people with primary, but normal, flat foot, in which case they lead to muscle wasting and weakness. The best kinds of valgus supports are individually molded and are made with a heel cup. This ensures that they are kept in exactly the right position. In general, rigid supports and pads are not as well tolerated by patients as supple or cushioned ones, and there is now a wide range made out of modern foam plastics

or microcellular rubbers.

The Role of the Surgeon

All surgeons would agree that the prevention of deformities in the joints of the feet is much better than operations to correct them. Much can be done for severe deformities but no foot that has had an operation is as good as a normal foot. The complicated balance of the foot and the mechanism of the anterior and longitudinal arches usually cannot be restored by surgery, and an operation to correct deformity may make another more likely.

For example, an operation for a painful bunion often results in a shortening as well as a straightening of the big toe. At the same time the surgeon frequently removes the small sesamoid bones — little pieces of bone that are placed inside the strong tendon to allow it to slide over the joint. These sesamoid bones form part of the normal anterior arch and it is on them that weight is taken in the normal foot. Removing them means damaging the arch so that although the immediate results of the operation may be good, in that the patient has a straight toe and is able to wear normal shoes again, later the results all too frequently include the development of metatarsalgia because of damage to the anterior transverse arch.

Similarly, the removal of a single toe because it is cocked up and rubbing on the shoe is sometimes followed by the other toes getting displaced into the gap and in turn causing trouble.

Therefore, if an operation is planned for the forefoot, it either has to be very minor or very radical — one that will not upset, or one for which it is worthwhile upsetting the whole balance of the anterior arch.

In the past the most successful operation for serious arthritis of the toe-base joints was to remove all the toes. This was a mutilating operation but it worked well and, of course, the feet could be hidden in normal shoes with a pad placed in the toe area.

Nowadays, more advanced operations have been devised that result in the toes being brought back into line. The patient can then wear a normal shoe, and something of the original arch is restored. There are variations on this operation, which is called forefoot arthroplasty, and in one of the most successful of these variations the operation is done from the sole of the foot. This means that not only are the patient's toes straight and the pain removed, but even the scar left by the incision through which the surgeon corrected the deformity is hidden.

Operations are also performed for trouble in the joints at the back of the foot, particularly if they are painful or collapsing. In such cases it is usually necessary to stiffen the joints, for it has been found that a rigid but painless joint is more useful to the patient than a painful movable one. The surgeon will usually put the foot in a plaster-of-Paris boot for a while to see if immobilization relieves pain. If it does, and if pain recurs when the plaster-of-Paris boot is removed, he may well recommend internal fixation of the joint by an operation. Extra care is necessary, since the patient with a stiff ankle is unable to point his toes. He cannot then get the foot into a normal lace-up shoe and shoes with extra long openings have to be provided.

Shoes and Appliances

Shoes made for deformed or crippled feet are known paradoxically as surgical shoes. Medical shoes would be a better term, since there is usually no question of operation.

Traditionally, surgical shoes are made using craftsman techniques. The craftsman or the fitter sees the foot for which the shoe is to be made; he measures it around the "waist" of the foot and at various other points and he selects a wooden last that is the nearest to the patient's size. He then tacks pieces of leather on to the last and by sanding these down and shaping them, he can turn the standard last into a shape similar to the patient's foot. The insole and the upper shoe are stitched together over the last. The shoe is then ready for the first fitting. If it is too tight or too loose, adjustments are made, after which the sole and the heel are stitched and nailed on.

This is a lengthy, time-consuming process. One skilled craftsman working hard can only make about six pairs of shoes a week at most. If the craftsman is also to spend some time seeing the foot for which the shoe is being made — as he should do — his output is even lower. It is therefore not surprising that such shoes are extremely expensive. In order to keep the cost down, the wages paid to these craftsmen are low. This means, in turn, that there are now very few apprentices entering the trade.

But the main problem now is that too many of these shoes are made by craftsmen who never see the foot for which they are making the shoe. The patient may have to wait for up to six months for a pair of shoes and, in the case of patients with arthritis, there is a strong possibility that the foot will change before the shoe is finally provided, so that it will not fit.

The traditional stitched and welted craftsman-shoe has another disadvantage. It is often very heavy. It dates from the days when lack of public and private transport necessitated walking, and shoes needed to be waterproof. But nowadays few people face the rain or the snow; they spend most of their lives indoors, in cars, trains, or buses. This is particularly true of people with arthritis. Therefore a much lighter weight shoe is adequate, and preferable. The patient with arthritis of the knees cannot afford to have the extra pound of weight on the feet that would result from wearing heavy leather shoes when very lightweight plastic materials would be more appropriate.

What can be done? In many cases patients with mild deformities of the feet can buy shoes that fit from commercial sources. Some firms make especially wide shoes for people with hallux valgus that is not too severe. They also make women's shoes that have ornamental lacing right down to the toes; this allows for a considerable degree of modification in the shape of the shoe. Some shoe stores now carry a stock of very cheap, light, soft plastic shoes which can look quite smart and do not press on bony prominences. Podiatrists can supply shoes that are deeply lasted so as to take a shaped or cushioned insole to look after deformities on the sole of the foot.

Also it seems that science has not ignored the importance of treating the feet. Many hospitals are now using a modern and effective technique known as the seamless shoe.

The seamless shoe is a general name for shoes that are made by bonding rather than stitching techniques; they are made directly from a modified plaster-of-Paris model of the patient's foot. They are derived from the so-called space shoes which were invented in about 1940 in the United States, long before the Space Age. The original space shoe made no concessions to fashion. It was a foot-shaped shoe, very broad at the toes and very comfortable, but rather hot and sweaty in warm weather because it was made of impermeable materials.

The modern seamless shoe starts in the same way. The patient has a plaster-of-Paris cast of the foot made. This cast is then sent to a manufacturer who fills up the cast with more plaster to reproduce the shape of the original foot. He then adds on extra plaster around the toes so as to make a shoe that is long enough for the toes to move forward during walking. He also narrows the cast around the heels to ensure a snug heel fit. The difference between the modern seamless shoe and the space shoe is that the insole material is now made of lightweight microcellular rubbers or plastics, already molded to the deformities of the patient's sole. The upper part of the shoe is not molded but is made of very soft materials which will not rub. Lacing is still the best way of closing the shoe, but for people who are unable to point the toes or whose fingers are arthritic and cannot manage laces, alternative methods such as a zipper and ring are available. Such shoes can be very light, weighing only five or six ounces, as opposed to twelve ounces for conventional surgical shoes. They can also be very durable — or at least they would be if they weren't put to so much use. The most durable shoes are those that are so uncomfortable that they are never worn.

Farmers and other outdoor workers who have foot problems can often wear their surgical shoes inside a large rubber overshoe or snowshoe. This gives almost as much protection as the conventional rubber boot and is certainly a lot warmer and more comfortable. Garage workers and other people who have their shoes exposed to oil have a special problem since oil and gasoline have a bad effect on the special bonding agents used. Under such circumstances the shoe may fall to pieces. It is necessary for them to be sure that special oilproof glues and cements are used in the manufacture of the shoes. Workers in machine shops where there is a great deal of metal filings have another sort of problem since modern shoe materials very easily pick up sharp metal fragments which work through the sole. Again, special care has to be taken. Such shoes need to be inspected daily and any pieces of metal splinter removed.

Given such precautions, the seamless shoe technique has been very successful. In one investigation, between 80 and 90 percent of patients fitted by this method were satisfied and were able to wear their shoes at first fitting, as opposed to the usual level of around 50 percent for the traditional surgical shoe technique.

11

Does Arthritis Affect Family Life and Sex Life?

Some forms of arthritis are chronic diseases persisting over many years and the doctor may have no alternative but to tell his patient to learn to live with it. And learning to live with a rheumatic condition is just what many sufferers do with extraordinary success, undefeated by what can often be a continuous nagging disability or, for some, a long-drawn-out pain. In fact, it is these undaunted people who are best equipped to teach and reassure the other, less confident sufferers.

It *is* possible to live with arthritis and rheumatism, to grow up, to marry, to make love, and to produce normal, healthy children. But it can be hard sometimes, and inevitably people worry about some of the real — and apparent — problems that they will have to cope with. It is for those people who need reassurance that this chapter is intended. The main areas of concern are how rheumatism affects:

1. The lives of children and teen-agers
2. Having a family and the methods of contraception
3. Pregnancy
4. Making love

HOW RHEUMATISM AFFECTS THE YOUNG

The Child

Serious forms of rheumatism in children are very rare. Strangely, very young children tend to accept it psychologically more adequately than those who are affected in their teens. A toddler or a young child with bad joints who has to go to the hospital and has to be kept in bed for a long time is often the center of a great deal of care and attention. Within the family he may get more of his mother's concern than his brothers and sisters who are well. At school or in the hospital, not only are there many people to look after him, but often there are other children similarly affected. He is rarely deprived of extra love, and the discomfort he is experiencing in his own body is, to him, normal — he has never known any other condition. The much-used saying "What you've never had, you'll never miss" is not without relevance to the child who has suffered from a rheumatic condition since infancy. If the disease persists (and only a minority of forms do), it is possible for him to grow up having spent a long time away from school, perhaps even having had many operations and treatments and having failed to grow to a normal height, but still feeling completely normal within himself. Such children do not appear to have any more difficulty than others in adjusting to the inevitable turmoils of growing up, but it is important for the parents to guard against causing the child psychological harm by being *too* solicitous and failing to make sure that the child attends to his own needs and wants as much as he can.

The Teen-Ager

The problems of contracting a severe form of rheumatism are more serious for older children and teen-agers.

For the boy, being unable to compete in games and outdoor activities can be seen as a catastrophe for his school and social life. It may cause him to become withdrawn and shy. For the girl, the belief that she might not be pretty may undermine her confidence, and some girls with rheumatism go through bouts of depression that are often out of all proportion to the apparent problem, just as other children go through agonies of feeling inferior because they have a spotty face or some inherited blemish.

This type of reaction is so natural that sociologists have developed numerous theories to explain it. "The looking-glass self" is a widely accepted concept which argues that people react in accordance with their ideas about the image they display to others. Thus, if a child *thinks* he is not intelligent, his work *will* be of a low standard. Similarly, a rheumatic child may become withdrawn because he believes he is not able to participate.

Parents and friends will do their best to help a disabled youth, but this can be self-defeating as it can create an attitude of reliance on others (and personal inadequacy) that could persist through life. It is better to encourage independence while simultaneously giving reassurance that help is available if necessary.

Sexual Development

The awakening of sexuality in adolescence is a complicated and sometimes painful process in any child, and children with rheumatism are not exempt from this process. However, the age when menstruation begins for girls and pubic hair grows on boys and girls, along with the other characteristic sexual developments for both, is seldom affected. And apart from a very few exceptions, their ultimate ability to become parents is not impaired.

Educational Development

For all children and teen-agers with rheumatic conditions there is a danger that they may miss school or training. Yet for them, education is doubly important — they may, after all, have to work with their heads rather than with their hands. So hospitals with special schools, schools for the handicapped, home tutors, and parents who will help with teaching and training are invaluable when arrangements cannot be made to keep the child in school. For children who have been severely afflicted, it may be possible later for them to be educated at universities or colleges that provide facilities for disabled students.

PLANNING FOR AND HAVING A FAMILY

Is Arthritis Inherited?

One or two rare rheumatic diseases are definitely inherited. The best known of these is hemophilia, the bleeding disease that also affects joints. Only men are affected but women who carry the gene for hemophilia can pass on the disease to their children.

Another very rare disease — ochronosis — is inherited. Children born into a family with ochronosis are unable to use one of the amino acids that is present in protein food. Instead, this substance gets turned into a black waste product that is lost partially in the urine, and partly is deposited in joints, damaging them.

If there is hemophilia or ochronosis in the family, there are special advisory centers that can provide information about the risks of passing the condition on.

Most other rheumatic diseases are not inherited in this straightforward sense, but particular conditions do occur more frequently within families than the average would lead us to expect. For example, in Chapter 7, gout was described as having a tendency to run in families, and yet there are more gout sufferers who do *not* have a relative affected than who do. Similarly, there is a tendency for osteoarthritis, particularly the type that affects the end joints of the fingers, to affect several members of one family. But the possibility of inheriting rheumatoid arthritis is very small. It is such a common condition that it is to be expected that, occasionally, there is more than one patient in the same family.

Family Planning and Contraception

The fertility of most rheumatism sufferers is completely normal. The only evidence of reduced fertility occurs in the uncommon disease called systemic lupus erythematosus and very occasionally in some women who have or who are ultimately destined to get rheumatoid arthritis.

This means that family-planning measures are just as important for rheumatism sufferers as for others. Mechanical methods, such as the condom for men or the diaphragm for women, may be difficult to manage for those who have crippled fingers. Most women with rheumatoid arthritis use the coil method (which has to be inserted by a doctor) or a chemical contraceptive such as the Pill. From the medical point of view, both methods are acceptable and safe, and will not make the arthritis worse or interefere with the other drugs used for alleviation of rheumatic pain. However, the Pill does sometimes cause aching of the limbs in young women, but it is mild. The aching stops when the Pill is stopped and it has nothing to do with rheumatoid arthritis.

Those who do not agree with artificial methods of contraception and who do not want children are best advised to abstain from intercourse. The rhythm method, in which intercourse only takes place in the so-called, and often miscalled, "safe" period, is not reliable. Menstrual periods often do not occur at absolutely regular intervals so that errors of timing occur; many unwanted pregnancies are a result of intercourse in the "safe" period. The alternative, *coitus interruptus* or premature withdrawal, is neither contraceptively "safe" nor psychologically sound and has little to commend it — it doesn't make good sex!

PREGNANCY AND ARTHRITIS

Pregnancy and Rheumatoid Arthritis

Pregnancy often brings about temporary alleviation of rheumatoid arthritis. Welcome as this is, it can be something of a fool's paradise — within a few weeks and sometimes even within a few hours after the baby's birth, the condition returns to what it would have been if the woman had never been pregnant. This sometimes leads to the pregnancy being blamed as the cause of the rheumatoid arthritis, when the disease had previously been very mild or unnoticed.

Interestingly, it was the improvement

during pregnancy that first convinced doctors that rheumatoid arthritis was a reversible condition and that research would one day find a permanent and harmless way of reversing it. A similar remission sometimes takes place in patients who develop hepatitis. Dr. Philip Hench postulated that in pregnancy there must be a Substance X circulating in the blood which suppresses arthritis. We now know that this is so, and that the Substance X is cortisol, a normal hormone and a form of cortisone produced in the adrenal glands. In pregnancy the mother is getting an extra dose of cortisol and in hepatitis, the liver, which gets rid of excess cortisol, fails to do so, so the amount in the blood increases. Unfortunately, this discovery did not lead to the hoped-for establishment of a total cure for rheumatoid arthritis. Cortisol and its many derivatives, of which the best known are cortisone, prednisone, and prednisolone, are only a way of temporarily suppressing this disease, and (see Chapter 4) if used in large doses or for too long a time, they produce unpleasant side effects.

Pregnancy and Back Pain

Back pain does not necessarily mean that the pain is arising from the back. Sometimes a previous disease or displacement of one of the organs inside the abdomen or pelvis (including the uterus in a woman) may be the cause of the complaint. So, because the position of other organs is altered when the baby is growing in the uterus, pregnancy may either alleviate or increase this type of pain.

However, pain arising from the lower spine is often made worse by pregnancy, particularly when there has been a previous episode of herniated disc or when there is a minor inherited abnormality of the spine. Special spinal supports or postural exercises may be needed to ensure that the whole weight of the developing uterus and baby does not have to be entirely supported by a weak back. It is easy to forget that although the baby at birth may weigh eight or nine pounds, this is only half the total weight of the pregnant uterus. Add to this the tendency for a pregnant women to put on fat and to accumulate fluid with swelling of the ankles, and it is easy to see why mothers with weak backs feel pain due to carrying around such enormous extra burdens.

Pregnancy, Rheumatic Fever, and Heart Disease

Happily, rheumatic fever and rheumatic heart disease are very rare conditions. But at one time, this was an important cause of death of the mother during pregnancy. In the later stages of pregnancy, and particularly during the birth process itself, the heart has to do a lot of extra pumping; rheumatic fever, when it affects the heart, damages the valves and makes the pumping action inefficient. The danger was such that in the past, women with bad hearts were advised not to become pregnant or, if they did, to have an abortion and, possibly, be sterilized.

Sometimes this advice led to bitter arguments, often on religious grounds. On the one side, there are those who believe that contraception, abortion, and sterilization are wrong and, on the other side, there are those who think that the health, and possibly the very survival, of the mother, must come first. She is not much good to her first-born children if she dies in the process of presenting them with a brother or sister. Fortunately, these difficult emotional decisions can nowadays nearly always be avoided. Birth can be brought on early when the baby is not so big. Operations can be performed to correct damaged valves, even during pregnancy. Drugs are available to sustain the damaged heart and to correct heart failure before it gets too bad.

Pregnancy and Hip Disease

Stiff, painful hips can make it difficult to part the legs and are a serious problem in pregnancy. A natural birth may be impossible and a Caesarean (surgical) birth will usually be needed. This is also true when the sacroiliac joints, which connect the spine to the pelvic bones behind the hips, are damaged. Their normal function is to enable the birth canal to expand to allow the baby to be born; if they cannot do this, the birth passage will be too small for a natural birth.

Pregnancy Relating to Other Forms of Rheumatism

Pregnancy does not make any particular difference to other types of rheumatic conditions, many of which occur long after the age of childbirth anyway.

But there are two conditions that are actually caused by pregnancy — the carpal tunnel syndrome and sacroiliac strain.

In the carpal tunnel syndrome the important median nerve which conducts messages from the skin of the thumb and adjacent three fingers becomes subject to pressure as it passes through the tunnel in the front of the wrist. Pregnancy can initiate this because it leads to a general increase of fluid in the limbs, which in turn can squash the nerve in its rather narrow tunnel. This pressure produces a tingling and burning sensation in the fingers which is especially troublesome at night. Fortunately, this clears up a week or two after the baby is born.

Sacroiliac strain sometimes follows pregnancy. The sacroiliac joints spread open under the effect of a special birth hormone produced in the body which relaxes and enlarges the birth passage. Each sacroiliac joint can be likened to the two parts of a scallop shell; because they are not smooth, when the two parts of the joint come together again, all the irregularities must fit exactly into each other. Occasionally there is a slight misfit and the pelvis tightens up with the joint in a strained position. A strong pelvic binder will often relieve any pain and should be worn until conditions return to normal.

MAKING LOVE

Even our Victorian grandparents, who would have found it difficult to discuss the subject of sex with any naturalness and freedom, would agree that if a principal purpose of marriage is bearing children and raising a family, then a normal sex life is essential. Today we go further and tend to stress the importance of a healthy sex life whether the couple desire to have children or not.

Do rheumatic diseases interfere with a couple's sex life? On the whole the answer is No, unless psychological factors interfere with physical consequences.

Pain and stiffness sometimes can interfere with intercourse. The most frequent position is with the woman lying on her back and her husband lying on top of her. She can experience problems due to difficulty in parting the legs or pressure on painful joints; he, problems due to the physical exertion involved. Alternative positions should then be tried. It may be better for him to lie on his back with his wife on top, or for him to sit on a chair and for his wife to gently lower herself onto him. There is a wide variety of such positions, and when there are some physical difficulties due to arthritis, it is important to experiment in order to find those that are most acceptable.

First, what is a normal sex life? Some recent studies of human sexual love have concluded that anything is normal as long as it is practiced by consenting adults. There is a great range and richness in attitudes toward sex among men and women. The frequency of intercourse, the time of day, the circumstances, all differ remarkably; for some couples twice a day is normal, others once a month or less; some are only sexually aroused in the morning, others at night and in the dark. Just as there is a wide range of what is normal with regard to frequency, so there is a wide range as regards preliminaries. Some enjoy an elaborate sex-play and ritual before making love, for others this is unnecessary.

Psychological Factors

Arousal is a psychological process even though it has physical effects. The signs of sexual arousal are obvious in the male, and although not so obvious in the woman, they are just as important since this leads to the secretion of mucus which is the natural lubricant in the sexual act. How does rheumatism affect the patient psychologically?

Significantly, 90 percent of the sex and marriage problems that affect couples where one or the other has a rheumatic disease are exactly the same old problems that affect non-rheumatic people. They are the typical problems that marriage guidance clinics deal with every day. They are therefore normal problems despite their immediate serious nature. Except in certain special circumstances, being a rheumatic sufferer does not mean that a person's marriage and sex life are bound to be failures, or even particularly difficult.

For the man, arousal is often quick but nevertheless dependent on a psychological feeling that he is a man, and this means more than just being a man in bed. It is not always possible for the husband who has a serious form of arthritis to carry out his traditional role as the breadwinner, going out to work to provide for his family. The sociologists' term for this type of situation is "role reversal." The wife goes out to work while the husband, because of his disabilities, stays at home perhaps pottering about attempting to do some housework. Psychologically, the loss of role can be difficult for him and may be reflected in impotence unless both he and his wife understand the problem.

An often successful solution is for the man to develop a hobby or interest, perhaps learning the skills of something he previously wanted to do but never had time for. One traditional function of hospital occupational therapy departments is the teaching and encouragement of hobbies for those who are unable to work or who are past retirement age. The wife needs to understand the psychological importance of these outlets and to encourage them even though they may mean more work for her on top of her already full program. Belittling the husband's hobby is to belittle him and may be reflected in impotence.

For the woman a psychological part of sexuality may be looking and feeling attractive, and if she feels attractive, she will be. Again, it is the concept of the looking-glass self; if she thinks her family — and everybody else — finds her unattractive, she will act according to that belief. Anything that may contribute to increased self-respect — such as attractive clothing, hair styles, and make-up — is important, and if she cannot reach shops and hairdressers, special arrangements to bring these facilities to her home should be encouraged — or better still, arrangements should be made to get her to them.

Surgery and Arthritis of the Hip

One of the welcome benefits of modern surgery for arthritis of the hip is that it permits lovemaking again. With a couple, one of whom has hip disease, this may make all the difference between a happy and successful marriage and one in which the couple is in danger of breaking up because sex is impossible. But even without the operation, lovemaking is still almost always possible if a position is used that the patient's arthritis permits.

Communicating from Single Beds?

It may seem to be a good idea when one person is in pain and having difficulty in sleeping, for the healthier member of the couple to move from a double bed to a single bed, or even to a separate room. But — and this advice is not meant to sound patronizing — think carefully about it; much of marital love is based upon good communications, being able to talk to one another, touch each other and to lie together. For some people the sexual act itself may not be essential, but sleeping apart may lead to isolation and to loss of contact both in the psychological as well as in the physical sense.

Some people find it convenient to make

love after taking tablets for pain relief. Others feel so stiff in the early morning and so much better in the afternoon, that it is worth any extra effort needed to enable the couple to make love during the afternoon. Still others experiment with the many positions and modes of lovemaking until one or more are found which allow sexual fulfillment for both partners.*

* Those who would like further advice on this subject are advised to write for the booklet "Marriage, Sex and Arthritis" issued by the Arthritis and Rheumatism Council, 8 - 10 Charing Cross Road, London WC2H OHN, England.

12

Spas and Spa Therapy

THE DEVELOPMENT OF SPAS

Spa waters have always been associated with the treatment of rheumatism and arthritis. The belief in the inherent ability of natural waters to relieve rheumatic symptoms is one of the few remaining indications of the symbolism that has surrounded water through the past centuries — one has only to read the Bible to see that water was often thought to possess magical qualities for healing both soul and body. In classical mythology, certain waters also had the same types of powers. For example, there is the story of Prince Bladud and the pigs who were cured of leprosy by the hot waters of Bath. But the use of water as a healing agent is not confined to legend. The ancient physicians, Hippocrates, Celsus, and Galen, are known to have used it, and as a more obvious example, the Romans built large centers with pools designed partly for treatment and partly as places for relaxation. In Britain, the remains of a Roman spa have been uncovered in Bath, and the pools and hot air chambers have been preserved and restored to an excellent state.

The Fashionable Development of Spas

Spa treatment, like nearly everything else, has been subject to whims of fashion. After the Romans left, spa treatment lapsed in Britain despite its popularity in the famous centers in Europe. It was not until the sixteenth century that Buxton became a fashionable resort for the nobility and gentry who came to "take the waters." At that time, treatment consisted of simply taking a quick dip in pools of hot mineral water and of drinking this water in large quantities. One technique reported was to begin with seven pints of water daily and increase this intake by one pint each day to a maximum of fourteen pints a day.

Bath only became fashionable as a spa center when the city was rebuilt in the eighteenth century to the magnificent designs of John Wood and his son. This architectural masterpiece, with its open streets, splendid crescents, and elegant buildings such as the Pump Room, led to the arrival of such nobility as Beau Nash and subsequently to development of the high status of Bath's society — as is depicted in Jane Austen's novels. As a result, Bath was probably the most fashionable center for spa treatment in Britain during the eighteenth century.

The Medical Development of Spas

But at that time the attractions of Bath and of all the spa centers were as health resorts, cultural centers, and places for relaxation rather than as centers for medical treatment. In some cities the original medical concept disappeared entirely, and today the recreational and amenity aspects are all that remain. In London, Sadler's Wells and Battersea Gardens are typical examples of recreational watering places that have lost their medical flavor.

During the nineteenth century, however, other spas became less fashionable and recreational and more medically oriented. Many centers endeavored to develop a scientific approach toward treatment and toward providing specific benefits for particular illness. Successful or beneficial treatment was claimed for many diseases which had little or no connection with rheumatism and arthritis, and the extravagance of some of these claims led to a more critical approach in assessing the value of spa therapy.

The modern spas were originally developed on the sites of natural springs providing water that had a high mineral content. The chemical contents of these waters have been analyzed carefully and were found to remain remarkably constant at any particular center. In some spas the waters are still hot as they emerge from the ground; this is due to some subterranean volcanic activity. Some heat may be generated by the decay of radioactive materials in the earth's crust. Fortunately very little of this radioactivity gets into the water that actually emerges.

The different kinds of spa waters — sulfurous, acid, or alkaline, potable or containing salts to the constituency of strong brine — depend on the nature of the underground beds through which the water is forced before it reaches the surface.

Do Spa Waters Relieve Rheumatism?

What then is the real value of these natural waters? Despite past efforts to prove otherwise, the claims that have been made for particular waters being of value for specific illnesses have not been verified. Nor does there appear to be any objective value in drinking the waters and in differentiating between the waters from different places. But even if there is no inherent healing quality in these waters, spa centers can provide the best sort of environment for treating rheumatism. The warm waters can be used for hydrotherapy and, more important, the actual atmosphere of the spa center is psychologically beneficial.

Psychological Relaxation

Spas are usually in sunny sheltered towns protected from the extremes of the weather. They are often surrounded by beautiful countryside and have magnificent parks and gardens with planned walks that will introduce the patients to splendid views. In addition to this, most spa towns, as a result of their cultural heritage, can boast of theaters, concert halls, exhibition halls, restaurants, and elegant historic buildings, which stand to this day and are still used and enjoyed. The psychological value of such a setting is obvious: the patient can make a break from the stresses and strains of his normal life — and just relax. Freedom from worry about work and home combines with the intrinsic benefits of spa centers to refresh the patient. When the physical treatments available in spa centers are added to this psychological relaxation, then the popularity of the spas becomes easy to understand.

SPA TREATMENTS

Hydrotherapy

Hydrotherapy is the term applied to the use of water as a means of treatment. This treatment is administered by physical therapists. Not surprisingly, therefore, physical treatment in the spa revolves around the hydrotherapy department.

The main value of using water — whether it is spa water or ordinary tap water — is that in it the body weighs considerably less. This physical principle was first enunciated by Archimedes when he showed that the weight of any object in water is decreased by an amount equal to the weight of water displaced by that body — which is the same principle that allows us to swim. In reference to treating arthritis, this means that a patient immersed in a pool need only exert a small amount of effort to support his body. Damaged joints can easily be put through a wide range of movements so that weak muscles can be strengthened. Hot water will relieve spasm in muscles and help them to function more efficiently.

Treatment is usually carried out in a large pool of varying depth so that the patient is immersed to the appropriate extent. The Hubbard tank is especially designed for hip problems: exercises are performed under water and the physical therapist can support the patient without having to enter the pool herself.

Exercises

It is in the restoration of movement and muscle power that the spas probably provide their greatest benefits for arthritic patients. In severe arthritis, the physical therapist assists the patient to move his joints while the patient is submerged in the warm bath. For the lesser and more common degrees of rheumatism and aches and pains, there is far greater value in the patient using his muscles without this help.

Local Stimulation

Local stimulation to the skin is performed by a wide variety of techniques to relieve pain in particular areas. A spray of water under pressure may be applied directly to the painful area and is sometimes combined with massage. Also used in some places are aerated baths, foam baths, and brine baths.

Massage

Massage is an adjunct to hydrotherapy and exercises, particularly for relieving spasm. It may be performed either in or out of the water or even while under a spray. But as the earlier reference to massage in this book suggested, its true value is rather doubtful.

Mud Baths

Mention of spa treatment often elicits the response, "Oh, that's where you get mud baths." There is a belief that different forms of mud and earth possess special qualities for relieving rheumatic pains. The reputations of the great European spa centers rested largely on this basis. These ideas have been fostered by the practitioners of mud treatment, but there is no evidence to suggest that it is any more than a useful method of applying local heat. These baths are prepared by mixing the mud with water and heating the mixture to the required temperature with a jet of steam. The patient lies in the bath for perhaps fifteen or thirty minutes and is later removed, showered off, wrapped in hot towels and allowed to sweat freely. Sometimes used is the mud pack, in which hot mud is enclosed in a bag and placed directly on the painful joint or on the back. Aesthetically, this seems much more acceptable. The combined stimulation of the senses by heat, touch, and pressure is particularly relaxing for muscles tensed up by pain.

Electrotherapy

This refers to the types of treatment in which heat is applied to the limbs with electrical apparatus. They are no-touch techniques in that the apparatus does not come into direct contact with the patient. By shortwave diathermy the heat is generated in the tissues under the skin, whereas by infrared radiation it is applied to the skin surface only.

All methods of local heating relieve pain — possibly because messages of heat and pain compete for the same nerves in the nervous system and these cannot transmit both types of message at once. The relief lasts for about half an hour after the treatment and this gives the physical therapist a chance to get otherwise stiff or painful limbs moving again without hurting the patient.

There is another way of using electricity and that is by a series of tiny (and not very unpleasant) electrical shocks over the nerves to muscles to make the muscles contract. This method is often used most successfully in teaching patients how to use muscles they have forgotten they ever had. The muscles in the feet are an example; they may need to be retrained in people with foot strain.

THE DECLINE OF THE OLD SPA

In the last few years the attitude of the medical profession toward spas and spa therapy has altered radically. Medicine is now seeking more direct evidence of the benefits of all forms of treament and of the positive value of any particular therapy employed. By and large this has been lacking in many continental spa centers, where many of the trappings used are merely holiday luxuries. But there are honorable exceptions, and some of the great spa centers in Europe have made outstanding contributions to the scientific study and the medical treatment of rheumatic diseases. Before journeying to a spa, the sufferer should seek expert advice on whether the spa is medically acceptable and not just a medically flavored holiday resort. In Britain, spas are being closed down. In Europe, spas are booming. In Britain, they are largely run by the National Health Service. In France, as in other countries, they are run by the government tourist agency. Could there be a connection?

For this reason, the influence of the traditional spas is waning. The disappearance of the spa is for many a sad farewell to an age of elegance which is no longer fashionable.

Although there have been great advances in the treatment of arthritis, these may have been at the expense of treating the patient as a whole personality rather than as a collection of medical problems. However, modern treatment centers are being developed in which the emphasis is on the specific medical treatment of the disease, combining drug treatment, surgery and physical treatment in one program for the patient as a whole person.

13

Acupuncture, Herbalism, and Folk Medicine

Arthritis and rheumatism have been described as diseases that produce prolonged pain. Most of the conditions described in this book are recurrent, persistent, and irritating; patients really do have to be long-suffering in the face of conditions that do not kill but for which there is no absolutely dependable cure.

THE SEARCH FOR HELP

Through Orthodox Means . . .

Treatment normally consists of regular, if infrequent, visits to either the family doctor or an arthritis clinic, but unfortunately snags can occur because of the very nature of these chronic diseases.

The initial confidence in the doctor — who can usually take steps to relieve the pain — may wear off over a long period of time in which there is rarely any evidence of a dramatic change or improvement. Patients may feel that the doctor is losing interest in them. Even more disturbing perhaps, in a clinic there may be the additional feeling of loss of continuity in medical care; doctors in hospital clinics change their jobs frequently, and so a patient visiting at six-month intervals may hardly ever see the same doctor twice. Consequently, each new doctor may fail to come to grips with his or her particular problem. These criticisms of our profession will — we hope — soon no longer be valid. In the past few years there has been a significant increase of interest by the medical profession in arthritis and rheumatism with a consequent improvement in the standard of medical care.

. . . And Via Less Orthodox Ways

It is partly this situation that has encouraged some people with rheumatism or arthritis to seek advice and help outside the medical profession. Any apparent lack of interest by the doctor in these persistent conditions is often fully compensated for by well-meaning friends and acquaintances, who may recommend consulting unorthodox healers or trying various natural remedies.

Folk remedies have been used for many different diseases. In particular, folklore thrives and flourishes in the type of chronic disease that persists for many years and varies in severity — such as arthritis. The natural course of these afflictions is not one of continuous and everlasting pain, but a changeable pattern in which the symptoms disappear and reappear for no particular reason. If folk remedies are taken and coincide with a disappearance of the symptoms, then whatever is being taken at the time naturally tends to get the credit. The big snag is that it won't work for someone else or even for the same person next time.

ASSESSING THE VALUE OF DRUGS

The problem of assessment of a particular drug or type of medical treatment is more difficult than one would assume. It is easy to be misled — many of the traditional medical remedies made no difference to the disease that they were supposedly curing or helping. Several factors can influence or bias an opinion as to whether a drug is useful or not.

1. The new medicine is not an isolated factor. Symptoms may come and go unrelated to the particular treatment being tested. To give an over-simple example: there is no known remedy that will kill the germs responsible for the common cold, but if a doctor said, "Remedy X will cure your cold in ten days' time," he could claim that remedy X was successful, for obviously you are unlikely still to have the same cold ten days later.

2. If an inactive drug is presented in a

positive way and the patient believes that it will do some good, this treatment is likely to make him feel better. This is the so-called placebo reaction: the new remedy produces an improvement purely because of the belief that it will do so — it is a psychological improvement. This reaction is precisely why witch doctors have been — and still are — successful in some parts of the world. Both situations encourage a self-fulfilling prophecy.

The psychological force must never be underestimated, as it can and does elicit improvements. For example, patients with angina or heart pain may be unable to walk more than, say, a hundred yards. But when a placebo is first tried, they may be able to walk double that distance before they feel severe pain. Unfortunately, this psychological benefit never lasts for very long.

3. The physical appearance of the drug is another factor that creates bias. Research has shown that the way in which the tablets, capsules, and mixtures actually appear affects the patient's response. Unpleasant-tasting medicines

are thought by some patients to be more effective than those that are either tasteless or can be enjoyed, even though the actual drug contained within them is identical. Even the use of different-colored tablets and capsules can provoke a biased response.

Nineteenth-century physicians seemed to be aware of this, for their policy — which was probably subconscious rather than deliberate — laid emphasis on the use of elegant preparations of medicines which in themselves were not very effective.

4. The patient's desire to please the doctor may influence his opinion of a new drug. When a patient feels that the doctor has taken a special interest in him and, instead of just leaving a prescription with the receptionist, goes out of his way to consult the patient and look for the most suitable drug, it is not surprising that he is more likely to feel that this drug is doing good.

5. Doctors can be equally misled when assessing the responses of patients. If the physician is enthusiastic, doing his utmost

to help, and is convinced that the drugs are useful, then he is more likely to see and record benefits for a patient who has been following his advice.

Today, the medical profession is fully aware of these difficulties of assessment and of the need for careful testing to make sure that new drugs really do work. The only way in which the true benefits of a drug are ascertained is by the double-blind controlled trial. This test is conducted by giving the new medicine to one group of patients and a drug of proven value to another group. Neither the patients nor the doctors know who is receiving the standard drug or the new drug and so the progress of the patients is assessed without bias. Both patients and doctors are studying the effects of the drug "blind." The key to who has been receiving which drug is held by a third party and at the end of the study the code is broken and careful statistical assessments are made to prove or dispute the value of the new remedy. It is only via this method that advances in the treatment of rheumatism and arthritis can occur.

FOLK MEDICINE AND HERBALISM

The double-blind controlled trial has never been used by the proponents of folk medicine or herbal remedies, so that the real value of their methods has never been tested scientifically.

That is not to say, however, that all of their remedies are useless. Many of the standard drugs used in medicine today were originally obtained from plants and have been used as herbal remedies through the centuries. For example the foxglove, or to use its botanical name, digitalis lanata, is an extremely poisonous flower which was given for centuries by folk medicine practitioners as a heart stimulant. William Withering then brought it into standard medical use in the eighteenth century, and an extract from this plant, digitalis, is still perhaps the single most useful drug for patients with heart failure. Similarly, an extract from the autumn crocus was, for centuries, the only specific pain-relieving remedy for gout. It is still used — in a rather more sophisticated form as colchicine — for gout sufferers.

But although there is always the chance that new drugs may be discovered from the actual ingredients of a particular form of folk medicine, so far most have turned out to be valueless old wives' tales.

Numerous plant extracts are used for folk remedies, but there rarely appears to be any rhyme or reason why one is chosen rather than another. The use of such extracts thrives on the belief that what is *natural* is also *good for you,* a belief which was as strong in past centuries as it is in the antipollution ethos of today. Just what "natural" and "good for you" really mean is hard to say. The wide variety of extracts used implies that they are of little help — if one or two were really useful, they would be used to the exclusion of all the others.

Apple cider vinegar is a popular folklore remedy for arthritis. It is based on the belief that somehow the acid helps to digest food and makes the tissues of the body more tender, thereby reducing stiffness. Interesting as it may be to speculate on this theory, there is in fact no evidence to support it, particularly as there is only a small amount of acid present in apple cider vinegar, and only a fraction of what is naturally formed by the body itself within the stomach. There is no possibility that this small amount of acid could make any difference to digestion or to the body tissues.

Those who swear by apple cider vinegar probably gain psychological rather than physical relief. A story to support this is that of an English devotee of apple cider vinegar who visited the United States — where it is the standard type of vinegar sold in the shops — and discovered that when it was freely available, it no longer seemed to be doing him any good.

Honey could perhaps be described as a herbal remedy of better taste. All the different types of honeys have their unique flavors (as well as being a good source of calories), but again there is no evidence that honey alters the course of rheumatism and arthritis.

Ointments and liniments are traditional remedies for aches and pains. Rubbing something in provides relief, but whether it is the "rubbing" or the "something" is unclear. Firmly rubbing in a liniment massages the underlying tissues and often relieves the muscle spasm that produces aches and pains. Liniments and ointments open up the blood vessels of the skin — producing redness or erythema — and this local improvement in the blood supply may be helpful in relieving pains.

Standard liniment remedies can be purchased from drugstores, but there are many herbal remedies that exponents claim to be more effective. Traditional materials recommended are camphor, dry mustard, and oils, but more bizarre concoctions that are supposedly used are made by dissolving live earthworms and ants. The results are no doubt quite magical.

Baths are used in spa therapy and certainly physical therapists know how to draw the maximum benefit from them. Folk medicine has also developed its own assortment of baths which usually consist of adding herbs to the bath water. Again, however, there are some bizarre ideas.

One practitioner has recommended the use of ant baths and even suggested applying live ants around the painful joint so as to bite the skin. Such treatment (in many ways reminiscent of sixteenth-century medicine) sounds rather more like a test of faith than profitable advice.

A copper bracelet for relieving rheumatism is probably the most popularly accepted myth. The misinformed argument behind this old wives' tale is that copper removes the electricity from the body. If a patient believes in his bracelet, then there is no reason for him to stop wearing it, but it is sad to see the clinic full of people badly affected by rheumatoid arthritis steadfastly wearing their copper bracelets — a fact that is evidence in itself of their irrelevance. A reason for the widespread commercial support for this particular folklore may not be entirely unrelated to the fact that these bracelets are made from copper costing very little and they can be sold at often-exorbitant prices.

Associated with the belief in copper

bracelets removing electricity from the body is the tenet that many present-day rheumatic problems are due to the wearing of shoes. Shoes, it is said, insulate the feet from the ground so that electricity is retained within the body. There are even stories of people who attach one end of a wire to the leg and trail the other behind on the ground so as to discharge this build-up of electricity.

OUT-AND-OUT QUACKERY

Sensible people, faced with the severe and constant pain of arthritis, may try anything to get rid of it. Some of these products may be harmless though expensive (frauds and rackets rob arthritis victims of over $400 million yearly), but others can be dangerous. Most important of all, these quack cures and remedies may waste valuable time during which arthritis may do irreversible damage to the joints.

There is no cure for most forms of arthritis, but real help can be provided. The only way to find relief and prevent disability is through legitimate treatment by a qualified doctor.

Since the quack's art is fraud, however, he can often appear quite respectable. The following list includes some of the quack's devices of deception. Beware and think before buying.

1. He may offer a special or secret formula or device for curing arthritis.

2. He advertises. He uses case histories and testimonials from satisfied patients.

3. He may promise (or imply) a quick or easy cure.

4. He may claim to know the cause of arthritis and talk about cleansing your body of poisons and pepping up your health. He may say surgery, X-rays, and drugs prescribed by a physician are unnecessary.

5. He may accuse the medical establishment of deliberately thwarting progress, or of persecuting him . . . but he doesn't let his method be tested in tried and proved ways.

ACUPUNCTURE

Acupuncture can perhaps be described as the Chinese equivalent of our folk medicine. It has recently hit the news in a number of fascinating reports which explain how this unusual system of medicine, steeped in Chinese history, is now spreading to Western civilization. Treatment involves inserting tiny gold and silver needles under the skin at certain definite points relating to the particular disease. This sounds unpleasant, but according to those who administer treatment based on acupuncture, the process causes no pain and produces a cure.

There is no scientific proof that acupuncture provides any positive benefits other than the psychological ones that are to be expected. It may be that the acupuncturists induce some form of hypnotic state in their patients so that at the time they believe themselves to be cured.

There is another possible explanation of how acupuncture might work. It is well known that soldiers in action on the battlefield may deny having any pain despite major injuries which normally would require injections of morphine. There must be some mechanism within the brain that prevents the sensation of pain reaching consciousness. This is the basis of the gate control theory of how the feeling of pain is prevented. An inhibiting mechanism is operated — the gate is closed — so that pain is no longer experienced. The psychological stimulus of a battlefield, rubbing the skin over a bruise, or stimulating certain nerves with the acupuncturist's needles may suppress the sensation of pain in this way. Operations are performed in China using acupuncture instead of conventional anesthesia, and perhaps this is how it works.

But both hypnosis and the gate control mechanism of preventing pain are essentially short-term maneuvers and can do nothing to cure rheumatism and arthritis. Faith alone in acupuncture often helps, but it does not represent any long-term solution to the problem. Carefully conducted double-blind trials have been undertaken to learn how valuable acupuncture is; several have now been concluded, and they failed to show any permanent benefit.

IN CONCLUSION

At first sight the rather extraordinary and sometimes monstrous methods used in folk medicine appear amusing, but at a deeper level it is sad that patients should have to resort to these measures. It is only natural that a patient should seek help for himself or herself. This is particularly so for sufferers with arthritis and rheumatism because their symptoms are chronic and recurrent, and although a lot of help may be derived from the types of medical treatment described earlier in this book, they may nevertheless be left with unpleasant symptoms. An understanding of the causes, processes and treatment involved in the various types of rheumatism is important to the sufferer — which is why this book was written — but a realistic account will give no unrealistic promises. Unorthodox remedies, often very expensive and presented in an elegant fashion, inspire a belief in their ability to do good. It is likely — and understandable — that these types of remedies will persist until the day comes when medical science finds a real cure for arthritis and rheumatism.

Resource Directory

WHERE TO FIND HELP*

Agencies

American Association of Retired Persons
555 Madison Avenue
New York, New York 10022

American Occupational Therapy Association
6000 Executive Boulevard, Suite 200
Rockville, Maryland 20852

American Physical Therapy Association
1156 15th Street, N.W.
Washington, D.C. 20005

The Arthritis Foundation
475 Riverside Drive
New York, N.Y. 10027

* The publisher wishes to thank the late Jerry J. Walsh of The Arthritis Foundation, New York, for preparing this appendix.

Canadian Arthritis and Rheumatism Society
45 Charles Street, E.
Toronto M4Y 1S3, Ontario, Canada

Family Service Association of America
44 East 23rd Street
New York, New York 10010

Home Economics Extension Division
(State University)

National Association of Sheltered
Workshops and Homebound Programs
1522 K Street, N.W.
Washington, D.C. 20005

National Association of Social Workers
2 Park Avenue
New York, New York 10016

National Council for Homemaker-Home
Health Aide Services, Inc.
67 Irving Place
New York, New York 10003

National Council of Senior Citizens
1627 K Street, N.W.
Washington, D.C. 20006

National Council on the Aging
200 Park Avenue South
New York, New York 10010

National Home Study Council
1601 18th Street, N.W.
Washington, D.C. 20009

National League for Nursing
10 Columbus Circle
New York, New York 10019

National Recreation and Park
Association and National Therapeutic
Recreation Society
1700 Pennsylvania Avenue, N.W.
Washington, D.C. 20006

National Society for Crippled Children
and Adults
2023 West Ogden Avenue
Chicago, Illinois 60612

The President's Committee on
Employment of the Handicapped
Washington, D.C. 20210

Rehabilitation International
219 East 44th Street
New York, New York 10017

U.S. Social Security Administration
Division of Disability Operations
P.O. Box 1075
Baltimore, Maryland 21203

Visiting Nurse Service
Consult your local telephone directory
for the nearest branch.

Benefits

Health Insurance Institute
277 Park Avenue
New York, New York 10017

Social Security Disability Benefits
   U.S. Department of Health, Education
      & Welfare
   Social Security Administration
   P.O. Box 1075
   Baltimore, Maryland 21203
         Pamphlets: "If You Become Disabled"
                        "Your Medicare Handbook"

Federal - State Disability Insurance and
   Welfare Programs

Workmen's Compensation

State Temporary Disability Insurance

Private Sickness and Disability Insurance

Clothing

Functionally designed clothing and aids
for the chronically ill and disabled

Vocational Guidance and Rehab Services
   2239 East 55th Street
   Cleveland, Ohio 44103

Fashion-Able
   Rocky Hill, New Jersey 08553

"Flexible Fashions"
Public Health Service Publication #1814
   Superintendent of Documents, U.S.
      Printing Office
   Washington, D.C. 20402 — price 20¢

Talon Inc.
   "Shu-Lok" Division
   43 East 51st Street
   New York, New York 10022
   *Manufacturer of "Shu-Lok" fastener
      for shoes; free sample on request*

Community Guides (for the handicapped)

The President's Committee on Employment
      of the Handicapped
   Washington, D.C. 20210

Easter Seal Society for Crippled Children
      & Adults
   2023 West Ogden Avenue
   Chicago, Illinois 60612

Diagnosis, Consultation, and Treatment

Family physician

Your county medical society

A rheumatologist
*Contact The Arthritis Foundation for
the names of local rheumatologists.*

Education, Information, and Schools

Local special school of education —
     board of education (for the
     homebound or the handicapped)

Talking books and spoken word cassettes
   Library of Congress
   Division for the Blind and Physically
      Handicapped
   Washington, D.C. 20542

Literature for the patient and the public
   The Arthritis Foundation
   475 Riverside Drive
   New York, New York 10027

"Accessibility of Junior Colleges for
     Handicapped"
A Survey by the Education Committee
of the President's Committee on Employment
of the Handicapped
Washington, D.C. 20210

"Careers for the Homebound: Home Study
   Opportunities"
   Pamphlet available from two sources:
   The President's Committee on Employment
      of the Handicapped
   Washington, D.C. 20210
   B'nai B'rith Career and Counseling
      Services
   1640 Rhode Island Avenue Northwest
   Washington, D.C. 20036

Employment

Federal, state and local employment security
   agencies

Bureaus of vocational rehabilitation

The President's Committee on Employment
      of the Handicapped
   Washington, D.C. 20210

The Governor's Committee on Employment
      of the Handicapped
   *Write to your state capital for
   information.*

Handicrafts and home businesses
   Small Business Administration
   Washington, D.C. 20416
   *Write for the "Small Business
   Bibliography."*

"200 Ways to Put Your Talent to Work
  in the Health Field"
National Health Council, Inc.
1740 Broadway
New York, N.Y. 10019

Homebound Services

Visiting nurses

Public health nurses

National Council for Homemaker - Home
  Health Aide Services, Inc.
67 Irving Place
New York, New York 10003

Homemakers — Home & Health Care Services
  Subsidiary of the Upjohn Company
  Kalamazoo, Michigan 49001

Meals on Wheels
  *This service is not available in every city, but
  where it is available, it is listed in your local
  telephone directory.*

Recreation

National Recreation and Park Association and
National Therapeutic Recreation Society
  1700 Pennsylvania Avenue, N.W.
  Washington, D.C. 20006

National Parks and Forestry
   Survey by the President's Committee
   on the Employment of the Handicapped
   Washington, D.C. 20210

Local parks and recreation departments

Rehabilitation

Physical medicine and rehabilitation
   department in your local hospital.

Easter Seal Society for Crippled Children
   and Adults
   *Check the telephone directory for your local
   chapter or write their national headquarters at
   2023 West Ogden Avenue, Chicago, Illinois
   60612*

Research

The Arthritis Foundation
   475 Riverside Drive
   New York, New York 10027

The National Institutes of Health
The National Institute of Arthritis,
   Metabolism, and Digestive Diseases
   Bethesda, Maryland 20014

Self-Help Devices and Equipment

American Hospital Supply Company
  Rehabilitation Products, 2020 Ridge
  Avenue, Evanston, Illinois 60201
    Large hospital and physical medicine
    supplier, several branches

American Velcro Corporation
  Dow and Canal Streets, Manchester,
  New Hampshire 03101
    Manufacturer of Velcro fastener

Everest and Jennings
  1803 Pontius Avenue, Los Angeles, California 90025
    Manufacturer of wheelchairs and
    accessories, gliders, ambulation
    aids, and reachers

Eversharp Pen Company
  45 Rockefeller Plaza, New York,
  New York 10020
    Manufacturer of "Clip-It" cutting aid

Fashion-Able
  Rocky Hill, New Jersey 08553
    Distributor of self-help equipment, including
    garments designed for dressing ease by the
    handicapped (mail order firm)

General Slicing Machine Company, Inc.
  Walden, New York 12586
    Manufacturer of "Vacu-Vise"

General Sportcraft Company, Ltd.
140 Woodbine Street, Bergenfield,
New Jersey 07621
Manufacturer of games for home
and institutional use

Handi-Ramp, Inc.
1414 Armour Boulevard, Mundelein,
Illinois 60060 and 58 Fraser
Avenue, Toronto 3, Ontario, Canada
Manufacturer and distributor of
fold-away ramp for steps and vehicles

International Business Machines Corp.
Armonk, New York 10504
Special program for supplying turned-
in electric typewriters to severely
handicapped at cost

Mars Optical Company
49 Bromfield Street, Boston, Massachusetts 02108
Manufacturer of "Reclino-Specs,"
mirror prism glasses

Milwaukee Faucets, Inc.
4250 North 12th Street, Milwaukee,
Wisconsin 53222
Manufacturer of Adjusto shower units

Minnesota Mining & Manufacturing Company
2501 Hudson Street, St. Paul, Minnesota 55119
Manufacturers of abrasives, adhesives
and cleaners

Ortho-Kinetics, Inc.
   P.O. Box 436, Waukesha, Wisconsin 53186
      *Manufacturer of spring-driven
      elevating seats*

J. A. Preston Corporation
   71 Fifth Avenue, New York, New York 10003
      *Distributor of physical medicine
      equipment as well as basic self-help devices*

Sears Roebuck and Company
   4640 Roosevelt Boulevard
   Philadelphia, Pennsylvania 19132
      *Firm carrying several aids for the
      disabled; shopping by phone service*

Southern Prosthetic Supply Company
   947 Juniper Street, N.E., P .O. Box 7428,
   Atlanta, Georgia 30309
      *Distributor of orthotic materials,
      Functional handle canes and Power Aid
      kit for motorizing manual wheelchair*

Sparr Telephone Arm Company
   R.D. No. 1, Box 241, Stroudsburg,
   Pennsylvania 18360
      *Manufacturer of gooseneck telephone
      arm to hold handset*

Spiegel's, Inc.
   1061 West 35th Street, Chicago, Illinois 60609
      *Firm carrying household, personal,
      and recreational items*

Talon, Inc.
  "Shu-Lock" Division, 43 East 51st
  Street, New York, New York 10022
    *Manufacturer of "Shu-Lok" fastener
    for shoes; free sample on request*

Vocational Guidance and Rehabilitation
    Services
  2239 East 55th Street, Cleveland, Ohio 44103
    *Clothing, mainly for handicapped
    women*

Wilhelm Jul. Teufel
  Neckarstrasse 189-191, Stuttgart, Germany
    *Manufacturer of portable seat for
    arthrodesed hip*

INDEX

Achilles tendon, 311, 314
acromioclavicular joint, 240
acupuncture, 388-390
adolescents, and rheumatism, 290-91
aerated baths,
age
    ankylosing spondylitis and, 45
    bursitis of the shoulder and, 242
    frozen shoulder and, 240-41
    gout and, 196
    lax-jointedness and, 254-55
    march fracture and, 309-10
    neckache and, 84
    periarticular calcification and, 223
    polymyalgia rheumatica and, 230-32
    pseudo-gout and, 220-23
    Reiter's syndrome and, 159
    rheumatoid arthritis and, 105-06
    slipped disc and, 8-9
ageing of joints See wear and tear
alcohol, and uric acid, 209, 213-14
Alexandra (czarina of Russia), 285

Alexei (crown prince of Russia), 285
allopurinol, 218
amino acids, 344
anemia
  rheumatoid arthritis and, 147
  Still's disease and, 274, 278
ankle (joints)
  internal fixation of, 330
  rheumatoid arthritis in, 314-15, 317
  sprained, 235-36
  See also foot (joints)
ankylosing spondylitis, 41-53, 157, 161, 164, 249
  associated conditions, 53-55
  cause, 41, 42
  development, 44, 47-49
  diagnosis, 45, 55
  persons affected, 45-47
  related diseases, 63-65, 88-89, 249 *See also* Still's
    disease
  research, 45-47
  symptoms, 50-53, 164
  treatment, 55-63
annulus fibrosus, 6, 8, 10, 80
antibodies, 166 *See also* immunity
antigravity muscles, 236
aortic valve, 54, 270
apple cider vinegar, 382-83
appliances, 125-27
Aralen, 140
Archimedes, 367
arthritis
  acupuncture and, 388-90
  in children, 256-58

disease-related, 263-81
    Still's disease, 65, 257, 271-81
  definition of, xviii, xix
  facts on, vii-viii
  family planning and, 344-47
  folk medicine and, 381, 382-86
  migratory, 266
  psoriasis and, 153-58, 284
  Reiter's syndrome and, 158
  treatment, 19-40, 94, 101, 188-93, 290-91
  veneral disease and, 159, 169-73
  warning signs, ix
  See also neck; rheumatism; rheumatoid
    arthritis; spine; names of specific diseases
arthroplasty, 189-90
articular cartilage, 177
artificial joints, 189-91, 280
asprin,
  for backache, 20, 164
  gout and, 209, 216
  for neckache, 96
  osteoarthritis, 191
  pseudo-gout and, 222
  for rheumatoid arthritis, 136, 138
  Still's disease and, 277
athletes, lax-jointedness of, 253-55
athlete's foot, 301
atlas, 80
autoimmunity, 166-67
automobile accidents, 85-86, 287
autumn crocus, 216, 381

backache

bone disease and, 7, 72-74
causes, 6-19, 29, 41-42, 80
inflammation and, 7, 41-65, 157
nonspecific, 18-19
pregnancy and, 349-50
prevention, 21-29
referred pain and, 42, 76-77
research into, 38-40
spinal structure and, 2-6
statistics, 2
treatment, 19-38, 251-52
tumors and, 7, 74-75
Bath, England, 362-63
baths, 121, 369, 370-71, 384
Battersea Gardens (London, England), 364
beat elbow, 243
beat knee, 243
bed boards, 22, 62
bed rest, 20, 33, 217, 238, 266
rheumatoid arthritis and, 119-23
beds, 21-23, 62, 90, 93, 120
bent-knee deformity, 117
birth control, 346-47
bleeding *See* Hemophilia
blindness, 274
blood vessel inflammation, 168
bone
diseases of, 7, 41, 65, 68-74, 289
impact shock and, 180
structure of, 68-69
bow-legged deformity, 186
bowel inflammation, 54, 161, 163
brine baths, 369

Brodie, Sir Benjamin, 159
brucellosis (undulant fever), 66
bunion (hallux valgus), 244, 306, 308-09, 317
   shoe-caused, 315, 317, 324
   treatment for, 308-09
bunionette, 244, 306-07
bursa, 241, 244, 314
bursitis, 241-47
   calcaneal, 314-15
   elbow, 243
   foot, 313-15
   hand, 245-46
   hip, 245
   knee, 243
   shoulder, 242, 245
   toes, 244
Butazolidin, 137
Buxton, England, 362

calcaneal bursitis, 314-15
calcium, 71-72
calcium gout, 221-22
calcium hydroxyapatite, 223
calcium pyrophosphate, 201, 220, 222
calluses, 308, 317-18, 324
camphor, 384
canes, 126, 193
capsulitis of the shoulder, 240-41
carpal tunnel syndrome, 245-47
cartilage
   articular, 177-79
   rheumatoid arthritis and, 109
   salt deposits in, 181 *See also* chondrocalcinosis

cell turnover, 209
Celsus, 362
cerebrospinal fever, 283
cervical disc, 85
    herniated, 85-87
cervical fibrositis, 87-88
cervical spondylosis, 81-84
    cause, 81-82
    persons affected, 84
    symptoms, 82-84
    treatment, 94-101
Chain, Professor Sir Ernest, 141
chairs, 25-29, 62
Charcot joints, 172-73
chickenpox, 165, 281
children, 339-43
    arthritis in, 256, 257-58
        prevention, 290-91
    disease-related, 282-87
    Still's disease, 271-81
foot development, 296-97, 302-04
neckache in, 238-39
periarticular calcification in, 223
rheumatic fever in, 263-71
rheumatism in, 256-58
    aches and pains, 258-63
chiropractors, 35-36, 99
chloroquine, 140
chondrocalcinosis (pseudo-gout), 181, 200-01, 220-23
chorea (St. Vitus' dance), 267-68
Clarke, May, 300
colchicine, 215, 216, 382
cold pack, 287

cold-sensitive rheumatism, 250-52, 261-62
colitis, ulcerative, 54, 64, 161-65
congenital dislocation of the hip, 181, 290
conjunctivitis, 160
contraception, 233, 346-47
contracture, 110
copper bracelets, 385
corns, 301, 307, 317, 324
cortisol, 348
cortisone, 63, 143-46, 348
crepitus (noisy joints), 185, 199
cryoprecipitate, 286-87
crystal gout *See* periarticular calcification;
   pseudo-gout
crystals, and joint inflammation, 198-201

dental treatment, and rheumatic heart disease, 270
diabetes, 172, 299
diabetic neuropathic foot, 320
diarrhea, infective, 159
diathermy, 371
diet
   backache and, 37-38
   gout and, 195, 207-08, 212-14
   osteomalacia and, 71-72
digitalis lanata, 381
discs *See* cervical disc; slipped disc
dislocation, 110
   congenital, 181, 290
diuretics, and gout, 209-10
doctors, and drug assessment, 377-80
Doll's flannel, 252
double-bind control tests, 380

dropped finger, 114
drug assessment, 337-80
drugs, as treatment for:
    ankylosing spondylitis, 62-63
    backache, 19-20
    gout, 209, 215-19, 381-82
    immunity, 146, 277-78
    neckache, 96
    osteoarthritis, 191-93
    rheumatoid arthritis, 135-48
    soft-tissue rheumatism, 249
    Still's disease, 276-78
dry mustard, 384
dysentery, 46, 169

education, of rheumatic children, 279, 343
elbow (joints)
    bursitis of, 243
    enthesitis of, 248-49
    gout in, 205
    osteoarthritis in, 185
    pseudo-gout in, 221
    rheumatoid arthritis and, 113, 116
electricity, discharge of, 386
electrotherapy, 371-72
Ellis, Havelock, 195
endocarditis, 267
enteritis, regional, 54, 64, 161-65
enthesis, 248, 249, 313
enthesitis, 248-49
enzymes, 200, 222
erythema, 384
erythema nodosum, 283-84

eunuchs, gout in, 196
exercise
    ankylosing spondylitis and, 55, 56-61
    neckache and, 100-01
    osteoarthritis and, 192
    pregnancy and, 349
    rheumatism and, 233
    rheumatoid arthritis and, 122
    slipped disc and, 10-11
    at spas, 368-69
    spinal, 31-32, 56-58
    Still's disease and, 278-79
eye inflammation, 33-54, 158, 274

fallen arches, 255
family planning, 345-47
fatigue, of joints, 179-81
females
    ankylosing spondylitis in, 45
    carpal tunnel syndrome in, 247
    cold sensitivity, 252
    foot problems of, 301, 303, 305
    gonorrhea in, 170
    gout in, 196, 202
    hemophilia in, 285, 344
    osteoarthritis in, 187
    plantar fasciitis in, 313
    Reiter's syndrome in, 159
    rheumatism in, 345-46 *See also* pregnancy
    rheumatoid arthritis in, 105
    slipped disc in, 9
    Still's disease in, 275
    systemic lupus erythematosus in, 168

fertility, and rheumatism, 342-43
fibrositis, 18-19, 228-30
  cervical, 87-88
finger (joints)
  gout in, 205
  lax-jointedness in, 255
  osteoarthritis in, 183-85, 345
  psoriatic arthropathy, 156
  rheumatoid arthritis in, 112, 114-15
  tendonitis of, 247
  See also hand
fingernails, 156
flat foot, 295, 311-12, 327
foam baths, 369
folk medicine, 374-76, 381-86, 390-91
foot
  bare, 299-300, 304
  blood supply in 299, 320
  development, 296-97, 299, 302-04
  flat, 295, 311-12, 327
  high-arched, 295, 312-13
  nerve supply in, 297-98, 320
  pain in
    back, 313-15
    front, 308-10
    middle, 311-13
  structure of, 294-96
  sweating of, 298, 320
foot deformities
  shoe-caused, 303-07
  shoes for, 331-37
  surgery for, 328-31
  treatment for, 325-28

foot (joints)
  arthritis of, 313-14, 316-19
  diabetes and, 320-22
  lax-jointedness of, 255
  leprosy and, 322-23
  osteoarthritis in, 186
  Reiter's syndrome and, 160, 319
  Still's disease and, 273
  syphillis and, 172
  wear and tear of, 315
  See also ankle; toe
forefoot arthroplasty, 330
foxglove, 381
fractures, 236, 321
Franklin, Benjamin, 216
Frieberg's disease, 310
frozen shoulder, 240-41

Galen, 362
gangrene, 299
gate control theory of pain prevention, 389
genetic predisposition to:
  ankylosing spondylitis, 46, 165
  gout, 345
  hemophilia, 284
  Marfan's syndrome, 253-54
  osteoarthritis, 345
  pseudo-gout, 221
  psoriasis, 154
  rheumatoid arthritis, 344-45
  Still's disease, 275
  See also inherited diseases
German measles (rubella), 165, 281-82

gold injections, 138-40, 277
golfer's elbow, 249
gonorrhea, 170-71
gout, 195-97
   acute, 203-04, 215-17
   after-effects, 204-06
   cause, 198-201
   chronic, 204-05, 217-19
   development, 202-05
   kidneys and, 205-06, 208-11, 214, 216-18
   persons affected, 195-97, 202, 209, 345
   psoriasis and, 158, 207
   research, 219-20
   symptoms, 202-05
   treatment, 212-19, 381-82
   uric acid and, 158, 198-201, 204-05, 206-11
growing pains, 258-63

hallux valgus (bunion), 186, 317, 306
   shoe-caused, 304, 306, 317, 324
   treatment for, 308-09, 333
hammer toe deformity, 312, 306
hand (joints)
   bursitis of, 245-46
   osteoarthritis in, 183-85
   lax-jointedness in, 255
   rheumatoid arthritis in, 112,
   scleroderma, 169
   Still's disease and, 273
   See also finger; wrist
headache, 237-38
heart disease, rheumatic, xxiii, 266, 269-70, 350-51
heart inflammation, 54, 266-67

heat therapy, 29-30, 94-95, 191-92, 133-34
  at spas, 371
Heberden, William, 184
Heberden's nodes, 184
heel
  calcaneal bursitis of, 314
  enthesitis of, 249
  rheumatoid arthritis in, 317-19
  tendonitis of, 247
hemolytic streptococcus, xxiii, 141, 264
hemophilia, 284-87, 344
Hench, Dr. Philip, 348
hepatitis, 348
herbalism, 381-84
herniated intervertebral disc *See* cervical disc;
  slipped dics
herpes zoster (shingles), 89
Hexenschuss, 11
high arched foot (pes cavus), 312-13
hip (joint)
  ankylosing spondylitis in, 59-61
  artificial, 150, 189-91, 280
  congenital dislocation of, 181, 290
  incongruity in, 181
  Legg-Perthe's disease and, 290-91
  osteoarthritis in, 186-88, 193
    treatment, 188-91
  pregnancy and, 351-52
  pseudo-gout in, 221
  rheumatoid arthritis in, 150, 362
  snapping, 244-45
Hippocrates, 196-97
HL-A27 (white blood cell group), 46, 165

Hodgkin's disease, 75
Hollman, Dr. Catherine, 304
honey, 383
Hospital for Sick Children (London, England), 263, 271
hot packs, 30, 94, 133
housemaid's knee, 243
Hubbard tank, 368
hydrocollator pack, 30
hydrocortisone, 36, 247, 249, 314
hydrotherapy, 131-32, 366-68
hydroxyapatite, 69, 199-200, 223
hydroxychloroquine, 140

identity cards, 145, 287
immunity, 106-08, 146, 165-66
immuno-suppressive drugs, 146, 277-78
Indocin, 137
indomethacin, 20, 62, 63, 137, 164, 191, 249
  gout and, 215, 222
infantile paralysis, 283
infection
  rheumatoid arthritis and, 106-08
    spinal, 65-67
  inflammation
    backache and, 7, 47-53
    crystal-induced, 198-201
    of the heart, 54
influenza, 227
inherited diseases
  hemophilia, 284-87, 344
  ochronosis, 344
  See also genetic predisposition

420

insoles, 326
instep, 327
intervertebral discs, 4, 15-16
    cervical, 79-81, 85-87, 89, 92
    herniated, 8-14, 20, 33, 36-37
        See also slipped disc
    spinal, 7-14
iritis, 53
iron deficiency, 147

jaw (joint), 185
joints
    artificial, 150, 189-91, 280
    ball-and-socket, 187
    Charcot, 172
    crystal-induced inflammation of, 200-01, 220-21
    early breakdown of, 175, 181
    exercises, 56-61
    fatigue of, 179-81
    incongruity of, 181
    internal fixation of, 330
    loose, 253-55
    lubrication of, 176-79, 194
    noisy, 91, 185, 199
    repair of, 177, 278
    research into, xxii
    wear and tear of, 174-88
    See also names of specific joints, i. e., ankle
juvenile rheumatoid arthritis.*See* Still's disease

kidneys and gout, 205-06, 208-11, 214, 216-18
knee (joints)
    bursitis of, 243

cold-sensitivity of, 191, 252
deformities of, 112, 117, 185
lax-jointedness of, 255
osteoarthritis in, 185-86, 255
pseudo-gout in, 221
Reiter's syndrome and, 160
rheumatoid arthritis in, 112, 117, 129-30, 163
Still's disease and, 272, 280
syphilis and, 172
knock-knee deformity, 110, 186

lactic acid, 209, 213
lax-jointedness, 253-55
lead poisoning, 214
Legg-Perthe's disease, 290-91
leprosy, 173, 322-23
leukemia, 75, 289-90
ligaments, 83, 296, 313
sprained and strained, 18, 233, 234-36
liniments, 192, 229, 383
longitudinal arch, 295
"looking-glass self" concept, 341-42, 358
lubrication, of joints, 176-79
lumbar corsets, 24-25
lumbar spondylosis, 14-17, 81, 174
lumbosacral strain, 18
lymph nodes, 274
lysosomes, 200

malaria, 139, 140
males
ankylosing spondylitis in, 45
carpal tunnel syndrome in, 247

foot problems of, 303
gonorrhea in, 170-71
gout in, 196-97, 202
hemophilia in, 285
plantar fasciitis in, 313
Reiter's syndrome in, 159
rheumatism in, 345
rheumatoid arthritis in, 105
slipped disc in, 9
Still's disease in, 275
manipulation, 33-35, 98-100, 241
Maori people, 195
march fracture, 309-10
Marfan's syndrome, 253-54
massage, 32, 95, 229-30, 384
measles, 165, 166, 174, 281
median nerve, 245
Medical Research Council, Rheumatism Unit,
(Taplow, England), 263
men *See* males
meningitis, 239, 283
mental rest, 119
metatarsal supports, 325-26
metatarsalgia, 308, 324
Morton's, 309
migraine headaches, 237-38
migratory arthritis, 266
mineral waters, 364-65
mitral incompetence, 270
mitral stenosis, 270
mitral valve, 270
moon face, 144
Morton's metatarsalgia, 309

mud bath, 370
mud pack, 370-71
mumps, 165, 238, 268, 281
myocarditis, 267

nails *See* fingernails; toenails
Nash, Beau, 363
neck
  exercises for, 58-59, 100
  research, 101-02
  spasms of, 239
  structure, 79-81
neck collars, 96-98
neckache,
  causes, 81-84
  disease-related, 87, 88-89
  nonspecific, 88, 90, 228-30
  related factors, 89-90
  symptoms, 91-93
  treatment, 94-101
neuroma, 309
nodules, 110, 266
nucleus pulposus, 4, 8, 9, 81

occupational therapy, 123-24, 357-58
ochronosis, 344
operations *See* surgery
osteoarthritis, 175-76
  cause, 175, 180-81
  development, 175, 182-88
  gout and, 204
  persons affected, 345
  pseudo-gout and, 221

symptoms, 183-88
treatment, 188-93
osteoarthrosis, 174 *See also* osteoarthritis
osteomalacia
  causes, 71-72
  development, 71
  persons affected, 71
  treatment, 73-74
osteomyelitis, 65, 289
osteophytes, 82, 83-84, 182-83
osteoporosis
  causes, 69-71
  development, 71
  persons affected, 70
  treatment, 73-74

Paget, Sir James, 75
Paget's disease, 75
pelvis
  enthesis of, 249
  infection of, 46, 164
penetrating ulcer, 321
penicillamine, 140-43, 148
penicillin, xxiii, 140-41, 171, 265
penile discharge, 160, 171
periarticular calcification, 223
pericarditis, 266, 274
pes cavus (high arched foot), 295, 312-13
phenacetin, 137-38, 312
phenylbutazone, 20, 63, 137, 191, 249
  for gout, 215, 222
physical therapy, 128-34, 192
phytic acid, 71-72

pillows, 22, 27, 93, 117, 120-21, 229
placebo reaction, 378
plantar fascia, 313
plantar fasciitis, 313-14
Plaquenil, 140
podiatrists, 324-28
policeman's heel, 249
poiomyelitis, 239, 283, 313
polyasrteritis nodosa, 168
polycythemia, 207
polymyalgia rheumatica, 230-32
polymyositis, 232
postural backache, 18
posture, 17-18, 90
    in ankylosing spondylitis, 44, 55, 61-62
Pott, Sir Percival, 66
Pott's disease, 66
prednisolone, 143, 348
prednisone, 143, 231, 232, 348
pregnancy
    backache and, 349-50
    carpal tunnel syndrome and, 246, 352-53
    hip disease and, 245, 351-52
    rheumatic fever and, 247, 350-51
    rheumatoid arthritis and, 347-49
    sacroiliac strain in, 353
pressure sores, 312
probenecid, 218
pseudo-gout (chondrocalcinosis), 181, 200, 201,
    220-22
psoriasis, 64, 319
    arthritis and, 153-58, 284
    causes, 153-54

gout and, 158, 207
persons affected, 154, 284
and the spine, 157
psoriatic arthropathy, 155-56

quackery, 386-87
quadriceps muscle, 129-30
radiotherapy, 63
Rasputin, 285
referred pain, 42, 54, 76-77
regional enteritis, 54, 64, 161-65
Reiter, Hans, 158
Reiter's syndrome, 46, 64, 158-61, 169
    after-effects, 161
    cause, 159
    persons affected, 159, 197
    symptoms, 160, 319
    treatment, 160-61
renal colic, 208
research into:
    backache, 38-39
    gout, 219-20
    joint disease, xxii
    neckache, 101-02
    pseudo-gout, 222
    rheumatoid arthritis, xiv, 117-18, 148, 152
rest *See* bed rest
rheumatic fever, xxiii, xxiv, 263-71
    after-effects, 266-71
    cause, 141, 264-65
    development, 265-66
    heart involvement 266-67, 269-70
    persons affected, 263-64

pregnancy and, 350-51
prevention, 268-69
St. Vitus' dance and, 267-68
symptoms, 264-66
tonsils and, 271
treatment, 265-66
rheumatic heart disease, xxiii, 266-67, 269-70, 350-51
rheumatism
acupuncture and, 389
in children, 256-58, 339-41
aches and pains, 258-63
rheumatic fever, 263-71
cold-sensitive, 250-52, 261-62
definition of, xix
fertility and, 345
folk medicine and, 382-86
hard tissue *See* arthritis
normality of, xix-xxi
sexual intercourse and, 346-47, 354-58
soft tissue *see* soft tissue rheumatism
spa waters and, 365-67
treatment, 367-72
See also names of specific conditions
rheumatoid arthritis, xxiv, 89, 103-52, 169, 241,
272-73
after-effects, 151-52
carpal tunnel syndrome and, 246
causes, 106-08
development, 109-10
diseases resembling, 153-73
fertility and, 345
in the foot, 301 *See also* foot; foot deformities;
foot (joints)

hepatitis and, 348
immunity and, 106-08, 146, 152
juveniel *See* Still's disease
outlook, 151-52
persons affected, 105-06, 345
pregnancy and, 347-52
psoriasis and, 153-55
symptoms, 110-17
treatment, 117-19
  bed rest, 119-23
  drugs, 135-48
  exercise, 122
  heat therapy, 133-34
  hydrotherapy, 131-32
  occupational therapy, 123-24
  physical therapy, 128-31
  splints and casts, 127-28
  surgery, 149-50
rickets, 71, 288
ring pads, 314, 325
role reversal, 357
rubella (German measles), 165, 281-82

sacroiliac (joints), 47, 63, 67, 157, 163, 352
sacroiliac strain, 18, 353 *See also* fibrositis
sacroiliitis, 63
sacrum, 4, 47, 68
Sadler's Wells (London, England), 364
St. Vitus' dance (chorea), 267-68
sciatic nerve, 10
sciatica, 10
scleroderma,168-69
scurvy, 288

sesamoid bones, 328
sexuality and rheumatism, 342-43, 354-55
    psychological factors, 356-58
shingles (herpes zoster), 89
shoes
    baby's, 302
    electricity and, 386
    foot deformity and, 302-07
    ideal, 307-08
    seamless, 334-35, 336
    space, 334-35
    surgical, 334-37
shoulder (joints)
    bursitis of, 242
    capsulitis of, 240-41
    osteoarthritis in, 118
    pains, 239-41
    pseudo-gout and, 221
    rheumatoid arthritis and, 129
    snapping, 244-45
skin conditions, 153-55, 158, 160, 168-69, 266, 274, 282,
    283-84, 341
slipped disc (herniated intervertebral disc), 7
    after-effects, 13-14
    causes, 8, 10-11
    development, 10-12
    persons affected, 8-9, 11
    symptoms, 10-13
    treatment, 20, 33, 36-37
Smith, Sir Grafton Elliot, 42
snapping hip, 244-45
snapping shoulder, 244
socks, and foot deformity, 305

sodium biurate, 210
soft tissue rheumatism, 225-55
  bursitis, 241-47
  cold-sensitivity, 250-52
  enthesitis, 248-49
  fibrositis, 228-30, 237-38
  generalized, 226-33
  lax-jointedness, 253-55
  localized, 227, 233-49
  polymyalgia rheumatica, 230-32
  shoulder pains, 239-41
  sprains, 235-36
  strains, 234-35
  tendonitis, 247-48
  tension headaches, 236-38
  treatment, 249
sole of the foot, 294
spa therapy, 132
  electrotherapy, 371-72
  exercise, 368-69
  hydroptherapy, 132, 367-38
  local stimulation, 369
  massage, 369
  mud baths, 370-71
spa waters, 364-66
spas, 361-67
  decline of, 372-73
  fashionable development of, 362-63
  in mythology, 361
  medical development of, 363-65
  psychological value, 366-67
Special Unit for Juvenile Rheumatism (Taplow,
  England), 279
spinal cord, 4, 78-81, 171-72

spine
  abnormalities of, 67-68
  arthritis of, 163-65
  bacterial infection of, 65-67
  degenerative disease of, 14-17
  exercises for, 30-32, 56-58,
  inflammation of, 7, 41-53, 163
  manipulation of, 33-35
  pseudo-gout in, 221
  psoriatic involvement of, 157
  structural change in, 7-19, 41
  structure of, 2-6
  supports for, 23-35, 349
splints, 127-28, 247, 280, 290
sprains, 235-36
steroids, 63, 143-46, 192-93
stiff neck, 238-39
Still, George Frederick, 271
Still's disease (juvenile rheumatoid arthritis), 65,
  257, 271-81
  after-effects, 276-77
  cause, 275-76
  persons affected, 275-76
  symptoms, 272-74
  treatment, 276-80
stimulation, local, 369, 389
strains, 234-36
strep throat, 141, 264, 271
surgery for:
  bunion, 328-29
  carpal tunnel syndrome, 247
  foot deformities, 328-31
  hip, 150, 188-91, 280, 358-59

neckache, 101
osteoarthritis, 186, 188-91
rheumatic heart disease, 269-70
rheumatoid arthritis, 149-50
slipped disc, 36-37
soft tissue rheumatism, 249
Still's disease, 280
trigger finger, 247-48
synovectomy, 149
synovial membranes, 109, 113, 114, 149, 315
syphilis, 171-73
systemic lupus erythematosus, 108, 165-69, 345
T-strap, 319
teeth, and rheumatic heart disease, 270
temporal arteritis, 232
tendonitis, 247-48
tendons, 113-15, 149, 247
   in the foot, 296, 298, 311, 314
tennis elbow, 248-49
tension headaches, 237-38
toe (joints)
   bursitis of, 244
   gout and, 203-04
   osteoarthritis in, 186, 193
   rheumatoid arthritis in, 112, 114, 301, 316-18
   See also bunion; foot (joints)
toe pads, 325
toenails, 318, 324
   ingrown, 301, 306
toes
   amputation of, 329
   deformity of, 306
   tucking in, 303, 305, 318

tonsils, 271
torticollis (wry neck), 239
total hip replacement arthroplasty, 188-91
traction
    cervical, 98-99
    spinal, 32-33
transverse, arch, 295-96
trigger finger, 248
tuberculosis, xxii, 66, 138
tuberculous arthritis, xxii-iii
tumors, spinal, 7, 74-75, 89

ulcerative colitis, 54, 64, 161-62
undulant fever (brucellosis), 66
uric acid
    gout and, 158, 198-201, 204-05
    production of, 206-08, 212
    removal of, 208, 216-17
    solubility of, 201, 210-11
    tissue deposits of, 205, 211
uric acid gout *See* gout

vaccination, 166
valgus supports, 327-28
veneral disease, 170-73
    arthritis and, 169-73
    Reiter's syndrome and, 159
vertebrae, 4, 67-68, 73, 79-81
vertebral body, 4, 73, 80-82
Victoria (queen of England), 285
vitamin C, 288
vitamin D, 69, 71-72, 288

wax bath, 133-34
wear and tear
  of the foot, 303-04, 315-16
  of joints, 174-88
  of the neck, 81-82, 89-90
    symptoms, 91-93
  of the spine, 7, 14-17 *See also* slipped disc
weights, in exercising, 130-31
whiplash injury, 86
white blood cells
  ankylosing spondylitis and, 46, 165
  gout and, 200
Withering, William, 381
women *See* females
Wood, John, 363
wrist (joints)
  pseudo-gout in, 221
  rheumatoid arthritis in, 112, 114, 127, 129, 149
  Still's disease in, 272-73, 280
  tendonitis of, 247
  See also hand
wry neck (torticollis), 239

About the Authors

Malcolm Jayson is Consultant and Senior Lecturer in Rheumatology in the University of Bristol, Bristol Royal Infirmary, and the Royal National Hospital for Rheumatic Diseases, Bath, England.

Allan Dixon is Consultant Physician in the Royal National Hospital for Rheumatic Diseases and St. Martin's Hospital in Bath.

Currier McEwen is a past president of the American Rheumatism Association. He was a founding member of The Arthritis Foundation and is a life member of its board. He was formerly Dean and Professor of Medicine in charge of the Rheumatic Diseases Study Group at New York University Medical Center, where he is now Professor Emeritus.